Disrupting the Intergenerational Trauma Cycle of High Conflict Divorce

A Guide for Mental Health Practitioners and Adult Child Survivors of Child Psychological-Abuse: Severe Parental Alienation

Volume One

Dr Alyse Price-Tobler PhD

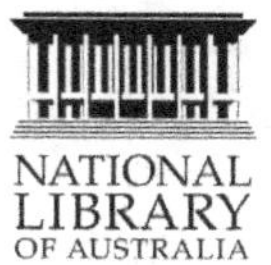

A catalogue record for this book is available from the National Library of Australia

This book is non-fiction.

BOOK #: 1

Publisher:
Inspiring Publishers
P.O. Box 159, Calwell, ACT Australia 2905
Email: inspiringpublisher.com
http://www.inspiringpublishers.com

National Library of Australia Cataloguing-in-Publication entry

Author: Dr Alyse Price-Tobler PhD

Title: **Disrupting the Intergenerational Trauma Cycle of High Conflict Divorce**
A Guide for Mental Health Practitioners and Adult Child Survivors of Child Psychological-Abuse: Severe Parental Alienation

ISBN: 978-1-923087-14-9 (print)
ISBN: 978-1-923250-17-8 (ePub2)

Acknowledgements

I want to take this opportunity to express my heartfelt gratitude to all the individuals who have supported me throughout my journey at The Sunshine Coast University.

First and foremost, I am especially indebted to my primary PhD supervisor, Dr Dyann Ross, and my secondary supervisor, Dr Peter Innes, for believing in my abilities to complete a PhD. Furthermore, I am incredibly grateful for the patience they have shown me as a mature student from a challenging educational background.

Special thanks go to Patricia Delaney-Davis, my surrogate mother for the past 30 years and the wise woman who has taught me how to heal my trauma and help others on their healing journey. You are an angel on earth. Thank you also to the universe and my family members who have passed for guiding me and keeping me safe. In particular, my great, great Aunt Dame Enid Lyons, whom I have drawn inspiration from throughout this journey. I pay homage to her and her words of wisdom when I think about the vulnerable people that I work with every day; "The problems of government were not problems of blue books, not problems of statistics, but problems of human values and human hearts and human feelings" (Henderson, 2018, p. xiii).

Thank you to my birth mother, Helen, for bringing me onto the earth to offer me the opportunity to try and heal our family's intergenerational trauma through my thesis. My heartfelt appreciation goes to my darling husband, Shane, for all of the time, unwavering practical support, and love that he has given me since the minute I told him I was beginning a

PhD. Thank you to my sister Kylie, my soul sister Dawn McCarty and my brother James for their staunch support and encouragement throughout this fascinating learning journey.

I also want to acknowledge my two beautiful, brave, strong children, Tristan and Alezandia, for their belief in my abilities and unconditional love. They have been my pillars of strength and provided me solace during challenging times. Thank you also to the beautiful, younger generation in my life, Lily, Rose, Isla, and especially my grandson Lyran, who was my inspiration and driving force to begin this journey.

Additionally, I extend my heartfelt gratitude to Dr. Craig Childress, a renowned clinical psychologist who has served as my clinical supervisor (for my private practice) over the past three years. His unwavering support and guidance in navigating my patients' challenges have been invaluable. Dr. Childress's expertise and mentorship have significantly enriched my professional development and clinical registration requirements. I sincerely appreciate his dedication, generosity, kindness, and encouragement throughout my journey, especially in helping me stay focused and balance my academic studies and work commitments separately.

Lastly, I would like to express my gratitude to all the adult survivors of 'severe level' child psychological abuse and the mental health practitioners who willingly volunteered their time, valuable perspectives, and expertise to contribute to my research. Their beneficial insights and willingness to share their experiences have significantly enriched the outcomes of these studies. Thank you for being integral to this incredible chapter in my life.

Dedication

I dedicate this thesis to three extraordinary men who died over eight weeks while writing this thesis between March and June 2021. The first was my mentor of 30 years, Noel Davis (1943-2021)- a quiet, gentle man who taught me how to trust and that people could be safe. Secondly, my beloved father, Geoffrey Charles Bonner (1944-2021) who died of 'unnatural causes'. I wish I could have the 21 years that were stolen away from us back every day. I love you and always have. Lastly, my beloved uncle, Denis James Bonner (1946-2021), was the funniest conservatorium-trained pianist I had ever met. You led a life as an outlier in society and are now at peace with your family. May you all rest in peace. I vow to fight to stop the intergenerational trauma patterns in our family for the sake of the coming children.

Sincerely, Dr Alyse Price-Tobler, PhD, University of the Sunshine Coast.

Acknowledgment

I have had the pleasure of knowing Dr. Price-Tobler professionally for many years, and I personally know her to be a dedicated clinician to the substantial benefit of her clients. Dr. Price-Tobler has a broader 38 year professional background in adolescents and adults with severe emotional and psychological disabilities affecting their lives, while also maintaining a more focused practice with the now-adult survivors of severe level child psychological abuse by a pathological parent.

The research and clinical work of Dr. Price-Tobler with adolescents and families in high-conflict custody litigation is superior groundbreaking research in a much-needed area, child psychological abuse prevention and recovery. The child abuse pathology in the family courts has gone unrecognised and neglected for 40 years of forensic psychology, as is typical for all forms of child abuse prior to its overt recognition. Child abuse is always a neglected and hidden pathology, until it is recognised. Once child abuse is seen, we protect the child. Until the child abuse is recognised, children are abused and remain unprotected.

The failure of professional psychology for the past 40 years in misdiagnosing (misidentifying) the pathology in the family courts as being something other than child abuse has led to generations of abused and untreated children, who now, as adults, struggle with a variety of life issues as a result of their undiagnosed and untreated psychological abuse as a child. It is to these now-adult survivors of child psychological abuse that Dr. Price-Tobler brings her research efforts to understanding their needs, toward a goal of developing a treatment protocol for the recovery of healthy development with the now-adult survivors.

Dr. Price-Tobler brings accomplished professional insights to her own personal experience as a now-adult survivor of severe level psychological child abuse and abduction in her own childhood history.

The life course that Dr. Price-Tobler took to her current professional accomplishments is a testament to the resilience of now-adult children of psychological abuse in overcoming both the psychological abuse of childhood and the neglect from the professional community regarding their damaged attachment beliefs.

Dr. Price-Tobler's research provides a valuable first step to understanding the unique experience of the now-adult survivors by a narcissistic-borderline-dark personality parent.

This ground-breaking research provides novel and valuable insights into the current experiences of now-adult survivors and potential insights into possible differing strains of the pathology's severity and expression. In particular, Dr. Price-Tobler brings potential directions for more deeply understanding the psychological damage to children caused by child abduction surrounding divorce and child custody conflict. Creating severe attachment pathology (psychotic-range) in the child for secondary gain of manipulating the court's decisions regarding child custody creates significant psychological damage in the child (from an induced persecutory delusion and factitious attachment pathology imposed on the child). The additional complex trauma of child abduction, however, adds an entirely new layer of trauma and psychological child abuse that the current research by Dr. Price-Tobler begins to examine.

The professional, academic scholarship of Dr. Price-Tobler is exceptional and is a credit to her mental health practitioner training, her lived experience, and her dedication to the well-being of her clients. The quality of scholarship from Dr. Price-Tobler clearly indicates her dedication to well-serve her clients and is a credit to the profession.

I anticipate with eagerness the upcoming Volume Two of her twin PhD study pertaining to the mental health practitioners who work therapeutically with now adult survivors, and additional work from Dr. Price-Tobler. Regards, Dr Craig Childress.

About the Author

Dr Alyse Price-Tobler (PhD) is a mental health practitioner/professional, lived experience academic researcher, clinical psychotherapist (MCAP), and the CEO and founder of 'Bowral Road Counselling and Psychotherapy Centre' in NSW, Australia. Dr. Price-Tobler has accumulated 38 years of frontline experience in mental health and disabilities work within the community. Her specialties include clinical-level trauma counselling and psychotherapy, academic research, and providing global support to targeted parents and adult children affected by severe parental alienation (SPA). In her private practice, Dr Price-Tobler's focus extends to complex-level private patients dealing with disabilities and severe and persistent mental illnesses, including intellectual disability, schizophrenia, bipolar disorder, FDIOA, autism, sexualised and criminal behaviours, eating disorders and dissociative identity disorder.

At the core of her unwavering commitment to research is her personal childhood experience as a child of severe parental alienation and abduction (SPAA). This experience has motivated her to embark on a groundbreaking twin PhD thesis focused on adult children who have experienced child psychological and physical abuse, with the aim of adding to the current research for the benefit of mental health practitioners (MHPs) and the well-being of future generations. Her seminal research is titled "Working with Adult-Child Survivors of Severe

Parental Alienation Abuse: Survivors and Mental Health Practitioners Perspectives." This innovative thesis comprises two comprehensive studies that delve into SPA support, treatment challenges for adult survivors, and the professional encounters MHPs face.

Dr. Price-Tobler conducted two concurrent rigorous research studies involving adult-child survivors of SPA and MHPs, specialising in working with survivors. However, these MHPs were not acquainted with the survivor cohort, a deliberate choice made to maintain the study's integrity. The study involved meticulous examination and comparison of data collected from two distinct cohorts to reveal nuanced patterns and variations. The primary focus was on understanding the perceptions of these individuals regarding the treatment they had received and the underlying reasons for their perspectives. This thorough approach is the foundation for developing a treatment protocol tailored to address the unique needs of individual adult survivors and their MPs.

Please note that Dr Price-Tobler conducted interviews with MHPs who were also international child psychological abuse experts specialising in parental alienation in adult survivors of SPA from around the world. In volume two, these experts present valuable insights into training, current treatments, and their experiences and perspectives.

Armed with a PhD and a master's degree in psychotherapy and counselling (MCAP), Dr Price-Tobler is at the forefront of pioneering therapeutic treatments for adult-child survivors of SPA. Through her extensive literature review, Dr Price-Tobler has identified a significant gap in therapeutic treatment protocols for MHPs working with adult survivors of SPA. Her work represents a vital contribution to addressing the pressing issue of suicide rates potentially linked to the absence of treatment protocols within this vulnerable demographic. Additionally, it aims to enhance the current standard of training provided to specialist SPA MHPs.

To connect with Dr Alyse Price-Tobler, please email
drapricetobler@sempi.com.au
or visit her LinkedIn
(https://www.linkedin.com/in/alyse-price-tobler-135459114/),
Twitter (https://twitter.com/AlyseTobler), and
website (www.alyseprice-tobler.com) for more information.

Abstract

Volume One of a two-volume PhD study provides new insights into the experiences of now adult-child survivors who endured intense custody conflicts involving court proceedings during their childhood. These individuals were subjected to severe psychological abuse by a pathological parent (Childress, 2015), a phenomenon termed severe parental alienation (SPA) in this research. This type of parent is commonly involved in family court systems.

Parental alienation (PA) refers to a process in which one parent, referring to the pathological (Childress, 2015) or alienating parent (AP), takes actions to negatively impact the relationship between a child and their other parent, known as the targeted parent (TP) (Haines et al., 2020, p. 3). This concept is defined as the APs behaviours influencing the child to reject the TP without a reasonable explanation (Haines et al., 2020).

However, in cases where survivors have experienced SPA, the psychological abuse toward them from the pathogenic parent (Childress, 2015) has been more extreme, forcing the survivor's symptoms to manifest to distressing levels and continue into adulthood. For example, children experiencing SPA abuse are adamant in their hatred towards the TP, refusing visits and even threatening to run away (Baker, 2007). They develop an unhealthy alliance with the AP, sharing paranoid fantasies about the TP, leading to the relationship's destruction (Baker, 2007). Some children experiencing SPA can exhibit extreme hostility, including paranoid delusions and baseless fears of being harmed or murdered (Gardner, 2008, p. 2).

The issue of childhood exposure to severe levels of parental alienating behaviours (PABs) is a prevalent and serious problem that can have long-lasting adverse effects on adult survivors. However, mental health practitioners (MHPs) are often ill-equipped to work with survivors due to limited training, professional development and the lack of an established best-practice treatment protocol to reference. Therefore, this research has investigated survivors' perspectives (Volume One) and the MHPs who work with them regarding therapeutic practice (Volume Two). In particular, these twin studies identify both efficacious and counterproductive mental health practices.

These studies utilised a research methodology involving a social constructionist thematic analysis approach and a qualitative research design. In addition, semi-structured interviews were conducted to collect data from eleven adult survivors and ten MHPs who were self-acknowledged as experts in treating adult survivors of SPA.

Survivors also encounter significant challenges when communicating their experiences to MHPs who lack sufficient understanding of the psychological and emotional complexities associated with SPA. This lack of awareness extends beyond social dynamics and underscores the need for comprehensive training and education across multiple domains for MHPs working with survivors of SPA, as described in Volume Two.

In addition to the hurdles confronted by survivors, these studies also document their remarkable resilience, given the profound trauma they experienced during their formative years. Notably, the results reveal that a significant proportion of the participants, as high as 90%, had achieved various professional and academic credentials despite their traumatic childhood experiences.

Furthermore, the survivors attested that their exposure to SPA and inability to find an MHP who understood their abuse had motivated them to actively pursue SPA information and resources for themselves. Additionally, during therapeutic sessions with untrained MHPs, the survivors hypothesised they had higher levels of knowledge regarding their child psychological abuse than the practitioner. These perspectives suggest that survivors have valuable insights to offer mental health research, conferences, and society stemming from their lived experiences and self-directed education. These findings challenge the prevailing narrative in current literature on SPA, which often depicts adult survivors in a negative light.

Also, the Researcher of these studies discovered three significant clinical findings while coding the data. Specifically, three of the four survivor participants (75%) who had undergone 'SPA and abduction' (SPAA) during their early childhood (under eight years old) described a potential new 'specific phobia, anxiety variant' to the Researcher that has not been previously researched or reported in the existing child or adult SPA literature to her knowledge. Given the limited research on the effects of SPAA on children under eight, this finding may carry clinical significance.

Additionally, it is worth noting that both phenomena are scarcely mentioned singly in the literature, so it is no surprise that specific phobias related to 'SPA' and 'abduction' have not been discussed together at length. Therefore, as this appears to be a new finding, the Researcher has named this variant the 'specific phobia-severe parental alienation, and abduction anxiety variant' (Price-Tobler, 2023).

In the unfolding of this twin PhD study, anomalous data emerged, revealing unexpected connections within familial dynamics. Specifically, the data highlighted a notable correlation between SPAA and other forms of psychological manipulation, including factitious disorder imposed on another (FDIOA), shared delusional disorder (SDD) and malingering by proxy.

As the Researcher delved deeper into the collected data, patterns began to emerge, indicating that participants who reported experiencing SPA also exhibited higher incidences of FDIOA and SDD within their familial relationships. These unexpected associations suggested a potential clustering of abusive behaviours within certain family systems.

Although the anomalous data was not intentionally sought out or investigated, its emergence provided valuable insights into the complex interplay of psychological manipulation within families. These findings underscored the need for further research to explore the underlying mechanisms driving these relationships and their implications for the psychological well-being of adult child survivors. While the anomalous data unfolded organically within the study, its implications sparked new avenues for inquiry and underscored the importance of considering the broader context of familial dynamics in understanding and addressing psychological trauma.

While FDIOA is typically associated with physical symptoms, it is important to recognise that some APs can also inflict psychological harm on their children, still falling under this term.

This type of abuse involves deliberately exaggerating or fabricating a child's psychological or physical condition with the intent to deceive (American Psychiatric Association, 2013). The Researcher posits that children who have experienced SPAA, FDIOA and SDD are more likely to develop the potential new anxiety variant described in this research. This condition has persisted in the study participants into adulthood. Additionally, 75% of the study participants who had experienced SPAA reported that they still struggle with paranoia and phobia as adults.

Thirdly, within the anomalous data, the Researcher discovered that, concerningly, 24 conditions described by six survivors in these studies were identified as autoimmune diseases or had links associated with autoimmune diseases. Additionally, the Researcher discovered that 22 of these autoimmune conditions were reported as having the potential to escalate to cancer (Sakowska et al., 2022), as highlighted in Table Five. Additionally, the figure of 22 potential links did not include the seven confirmed cancer conditions collected from 1 MHP's data (Volume Two), as this figure is speculative. However, when the Researcher added all of the figures from the previous research and these studies, adult survivors and MHPs might be susceptible to 39 autoimmune diseases and 35 different types of cancer.

Important note: In discussing the previously described data in these studies, it is important to acknowledge certain caveats. Firstly, the Researcher reports that the information presented represents the survivors' perspectives from these studies. Additionally, the Researcher has investigated potential links to autoimmune disease and cancer from other peer-reviewed studies and compared the data to this research. It is crucial to recognise that data from these studies may not have reached the level of support typically expected in rigorous research. However, it serves as a valuable starting point for future investigations to build upon.

These studies present valuable insights into adult survivors of child psychological abuse in addressing the challenges of SPA support and treatment. They also emphasise the need for further research and professional development in treating SPA and the associated CITs. Equipping MHPs with knowledge and tools is crucial to support survivors effectively.

These findings lay the groundwork for clinical trials to develop a new evidence-based treatment protocol for adult survivors. Additionally, the Researcher is currently developing the protocol. In conclusion, the findings of these studies underscore the urgent need for action to recognise and address the unique and complex needs of adult-child survivors of severe child psychological abuse.

Table of Contents

List of Figures

List of Tables

Please note: Due to the restructuring necessitated by removing chapters from Volume One into Volume Two, some sequencing of the 'Tables' has been disrupted, resulting in an irregular flow. Please refer to Volume Two, 'Mental Health Practitioners', for the missing Tables as required.

List of Appendices

Abbreviations and Acronyms

Acronyms	
ABPA	Attachment-Based Parental Alienation
ACES	Adverse Childhood Experiences
ACE's	Adverse Childhood Experiences Study
BSQ	Baker Strategy Questionnaire
CITs	Complex Intersecting Traumas
CSA	Child Sexual Abuse
CTT	Contemporary Trauma Theory
FDIOA	Factitious Disorder Imposed On Another
FDV	Family and Domestic Violence
IPV	Intimate Partner Violence
MH	Mental Health
MHP	Mental Health Practitioner
MHPs	Mental Health Practitioners
MRSA	Methicillin-resistant Staphylococcus aureus

PA	Parental Alienation
PABs	Parental Alienating Behaviours
PAS	Parental Alienation Syndrome
SPA	Severe Parental Alienation
SPAA	Severe Parental Alienation and Abduction
TIC	Trauma Informed Care

Please note that abbreviations and acronyms that were only mentioned once or twice were not included in this table.

Statement of Original Authorship

This thesis *is composed of my original work and contains* no material previously published or written by another person except where due reference has been made in the text. I have not engaged an editor to help me with this thesis.

I have clearly stated the contribution of others to my thesis as a whole, including statistical assistance, survey design, data analysis, significant technical procedures, professional editorial advice, financial support and any other original research work used or reported in my thesis. The content of my thesis is the result of work I have carried out since the commencement of my higher degree by research candidature and does not include a substantial part of work that has been submitted *to qualify for the award of any* other degree or diploma in any university or other tertiary institution. I have clearly stated which parts of my thesis, if any, have been submitted to qualify for another award.

I acknowledge that an electronic copy of my thesis must be lodged with the University Library and, subject to the policy and procedures of The University of the Sunshine Coast, the thesis be made available for research and study in accordance with the Copyright Act 1968 unless a period of embargo has been approved by the Dean of Graduate Research.

I acknowledge that the copyright of all material contained in my thesis resides with the copyright holder(s) of that material. Where appropriate, I have obtained copyright permission from the copyright holder to reproduce material in this thesis and have sought permission from co-authors for any jointly authored works included in the thesis.

Finally, this thesis was solely prepared and edited by the author. No professional editors or external assistants were involved in this work's writing, editing, or content development.

Alyse Price-Tobler 18.8.23

Financial Support

I also acknowledge that this research was supported by an Australian Government Research Training Program Scholarship, which I deeply appreciate for its contribution to the realisation of this research endeavour.

Ethics Approval for Research

Human research ethics approval for the research project: Working with Adult Survivors of Severe Parental Alienation: Survivors and Mental Health Practitioners Perspectives. A Qualitative Study (S211642).

Human subjects were involved in this research.

The Researcher applied for and was granted ethics approval with the University of the Sunshine Coast to follow appropriate scientific protocol. Ethical clearance was obtained from the National Health and Medical Research Council (NHMRC) through the Human Research Ethics Application (HREA), approval number S211642.

A letter of approval was sent on December 21, 2021, by A/Prof Andrew Crowden, Chair, Human Research Ethics Committee Tel: +61 7 5430 2823 Email: humanethics@usc.edu.au

The letter of approval is included in Appendix Ten.

Introduction

The twin PhD thesis reveals the prevalence of childhood exposure to severe parental alienation behaviours (PABs), which can have enduring adverse effects on adult survivors. Moreover, it highlights the lack of training or awareness among MHPs on effectively supporting adult survivors of SPA. The first volume of the thesis gathers the perspectives of adult survivors who have accessed treatment involving their child psychological and physical abuse- severe parental alienation, as discerned from their perspectives. These survivors provide valuable insights and advice on improving collaboration with MHPs who support them.

Method

This research aimed to explore the perspectives and needs of adult survivors of SPA (volume one) when engaging in therapy to identify helpful and unhelpful mental health practices. This study used a qualitative approach, gathering data through semi-structured interviews and evaluating it via thematic analysis guided by a social constructionist epistemology. Eleven survivors of SPA and ten MHP experts (volume two) specialising in child psychological and physical abuse- severe parental alienation participated in the study.

Results Pertaining to Adult Survivors

The study found that survivors experience significant difficulties explaining their experiences to MHPs who lack a thorough understanding of SPA's psychological, physical and social dimensions. The study's findings also report adverse psychological, physical and social implications for MHPs who work with adult child survivors of SPA, which is reported in volume two.

Significantly, the research reveals a substantial link between autoimmune diseases and cancer, with potential implications for both survivors and MHPs. The study uncovers that 24 conditions reported by survivors are identified as autoimmune diseases or have associated links. Of these, 22 autoimmune conditions are reported as having the potential to escalate to cancer. While the figure of 22 potential links does not include the seven confirmed cancer conditions from one MHP's data, it implies that adult survivors and MHPs could potentially be at risk for 39 autoimmune diseases and 35 different types of cancer.

The article emphasises the need for interdisciplinary collaboration to comprehensively address these complex issues and enhance support for survivors and MHPs. It is important to note that this article incorporates data from these studies and three prior research reports, laying a critical foundation for understanding potential associations between autoimmune diseases and cancer among SPA survivors and MHPs.

However, certain caveats must be acknowledged. While the research highlights the potential links between autoimmune diseases and cancer, it primarily falls within the domain of psychology. The data collected, though rigorously examined, may not meet the typical standards of medical research. The thesis serves as an essential starting point for future investigations in this uncharted territory of SPA survivors' health.

Dr Price-Tobler also reported discovering two significant clinical findings while coding the data. Specifically, three of the four survivor participants (75%) who had undergone 'SPA and abduction' (SPAA) during their early childhood (under six years old) described a 'specific phobia, anxiety variant' to the Researcher that has not been previously researched or reported in the existing child or adult SPA literature. Given the limited research on the effects of 'SPA and abduction' on children under six, this finding carries clinical significance.

Additionally, it is worth noting that both phenomena are scarcely mentioned singly in the literature, so it is no surprise that specific phobias related to 'SPA' and 'abduction' have not been discussed together at length. Furthermore, there is a dearth of information when these terms are directly connected. Therefore, as this seems to be a new finding, the Researcher has named this variant the "specific phobia-severe parental alienation, and abduction anxiety variant" (Price-Tobler, 2023).

In addition to the challenges faced by survivors of SPA, the study also found that survivors exhibited high levels of resilience and had achieved over twenty university and professional degrees, double the survivor study participant number. Furthermore, survivors reported that their experiences of SPA had led them to seek out information and resources independently. Many referred to themselves as self-taught experts in the area of SPA, often claiming that they knew more than the practitioner they were seeking therapy from. These findings suggest that adult survivors of SPA have the potential to make significant contributions to the field of society and mental health psychology.

Finally, practitioners will benefit from this study's results by acknowledging and understanding how survivors gain resilience and knowledge to help themselves heal. This study's results suggest that practitioners must take a collaborative, holistic, and respectful approach when working with survivors, particularly those who belong to vulnerable groups such as Indigenous Australians and African Americans while valuing survivors' lived experience perspectives and insights.

Overall, this twin PhD thesis provides valuable insights into adult survivors of SPA and the perspectives of their experiences with the MHPs who work with them. The study highlights the need for more research and professional development in the area of adult survivors of SPA and the importance of providing MHPs with the tools and knowledge they need to support themselves and survivors holistically, safely and effectively. This study makes a significant contribution to the mental health profession. Its findings illuminate a previously under-researched area and offer innovative insights for both adult children of child psychological and physical abuse- SPA and their MHPs. By addressing the most pressing concerns of adult survivors of SPA and their practitioners, this thesis enriches our understanding of the effects of SPA on adult-child survivors, providing valuable knowledge to the field.

Chapter One

Background

In 1969, Governor Ronald Reagan of California, USA, made what he called one of the biggest mistakes of his political life (Wilcox, 2009). Seeking to eliminate the deception and conflict associated with the legal system of fault-based divorce, Reagan signed America's first no-fault divorce bill. The new law gave couples the go-ahead to pursue a divorce without proving any fault on either side, essentially gutting marriage and its legal power to bind together a husband and wife (Wilcox, 2009). Paul Amato (n.d) estimates that if the United States of America maintained their family levels of stability, much like in the 1960s, there would be approximately 70,000 fewer suicide attempts every year (Wilcox, 2009).

Currently, 3.8 million children are suspected of experiencing moderate to child psychological abuse, also known as parental alienation (PA) by one of their parents in America in 2019 (Harman et al., 2019). In addition, in 2014, the divorce industry was estimated to be worth 50 billion dollars annually in the US (MCMoewe, 2014). In Australia in 2019, 113,815 marriages were registered with the Australian Bureau of Statistics (2020), and 49,116 divorces were granted (Australian Government, 2019). Also, in 2019, 2,015,603 marriages were recorded in America and 746,971 divorces (Centers for Disease Control and Prevention, 2020).

Furthermore, historical research reports that there were 100,000 custody battles taking place in the United States of America and that these disputes were generally hostile and stressful (Turkat, 2000). Over the past two decades, the statistics surrounding divorcing families, the prevalence of SPA experienced by children and adolescents, and the financial implications of divorce have undergone unprecedented changes. However, current research on child psychological abuse, aka severe parental alienation (SPA), has primarily concentrated on children and adolescents affected by divorce and custody disputes rather than examining the experiences of survivors of divorce, PA, or SPA. Parental alienation (PA) refers to a process in which one parent (referring to the alienating parent or AP) takes actions to negatively impact the relationship between a child and their other parent (known as the targeted parent or TP) (Haines et al., 2020, p. 3). This concept is defined as the alienating parents' behaviours influencing the child to reject the TP without a reasonable explanation (Haines et al., 2020). Such behaviours cause significant harm to the child's relationship with their TP. It is important to note that PA is distinct from situations involving reasonable rejection, abuse, compromised parenting, or genuine estrangement of a parent due to neglect (Fidler et al., 2012). For example, parental estrangement is defined as a child rejecting a parent for a genuine reason, such as a substantiated history of neglect, abuse, or severely inadequate parenting (Lorandos & Bernet, 2020).

Noted psychiatrist and controversial early PA researcher Richard Gardner (1998) explains that PA occurs during a post-divorce custody arrangement when one parent successfully manipulates the child to turn against the other parent. This manipulation can range from subtle behaviours to overt actions, such as making false allegations of physical or sexual abuse or denying contact with the TP.

Clinical Definition of Parental Alienation

At a clinical level, adult child psychological abuse, also known as "parental alienation", involves a child getting drawn into their parents' marital conflict by forming a coalition with a narcissistic or borderline parent against the other parent (Childress, 2015). This alliance leads to a breakdown in the child's relationship with the TP (Childress, 2015). The narcissistic or borderline parent uses the child to manage their own anxiety stemming from the divorce, essentially reversing the parent-child roles to ease their distress (Childress, 2015). This anxiety arises from three main sources: narcissistic anxiety, which threatens the parent's self-image; borderline anxiety, rooted in fear of abandonment; and trauma anxiety, linked to unresolved childhood attachment issues driving parental alienation (Childress, 2015).

However, continually referring to this clinical phenomenon by its full definition can be cumbersome. Alternative terms like "trauma reenactment alienation" or "induced child rejection through role reversal" have been suggested, but "parental alienation" remains the commonly used term. While not a precise clinical term, "parental alienation" encompasses a range of clinical constructs with defined meanings in scientific literature.

Please note that adult-child psychological abuse will be referred to as "parental alienation" throughout this book due to the general public being more familiar with this term.

The effects of SPA can be highly detrimental, often resulting in children displaying behavioural difficulties such as anxiety, depression, and low self-esteem (Baker, 2007). In addition, such forms of abuse frequently contribute to long-lasting psychological and social issues during adulthood. For instance, in cases of SPA, children commonly express feelings of fear and intense dislike towards the TP, steadfastly refusing to establish any form of relationship with them. APs will use tactics aimed at the child to increase dependence on them and away from the TP (Lorandos & Bernet, 2020). These tactics are described by Giancarlo (2019) as starting to withhold love if a child directs affection toward the TP, imparting fear in a child, exhibiting non-compliance with court orders, interference with the child's phone contacts or emails, or seeking restraining orders for unfounded allegations. PA tactics also involve a campaign of denigration led by one parent that consists of the child as unknowing and later as a knowing participant. Later, they may join the AP against the TP to demolish any relationship between the TP and themselves (Bernet, 2008). Thus, within the PA dynamic, the targeted and now alienated parent is placed in a position where they are constantly required to placate the AP to maintain a relationship with their child (Giancarlo, 2019). Tactics are further described in "Three Types of Alienating Parents" (Bernet, 2010).

PA Terminology

The PA terminology and definitions used by some researchers referenced in the study use language that may be misconstrued as violent communication. For example, Rosenberg (2015, p. 15) explains that "certain ways of communicating alienate us from our natural state of compassion". For example, Rosenberg (2015, p. 15) states,

> Life-alienating communication traps us in a world of judgments, using language that classifies and divides people based on rightness and wrongness. We constantly judge others, labelling them as good, bad, normal, abnormal, responsible, irresponsible, smart, ignorant, and more (Rosenberg, 2015).

A person-centred approach, rather than a disorder-focused approach to understanding SPA trauma sequelae, was drawn upon during the interview process for these studies. A person-centred approach is described as supporting a person in being involved in their decision-making regarding their life and considering their life experience (NSW Government Health, 2020). Factors that come into consideration include a person's gender, age, heritage, culture, identity, beliefs, and language (NSW Government Health, 2020). The person-centred approach is a strengths-based method where people are acknowledged as experts in their own lives, focusing on what actions they can complete for themselves, followed by the identification of needing help from others (NSW Government Health, 2020).

The terminology review aims to discern the most appropriate language for the research, thereby avoiding the constructions of people in potentially harmful or violent ways. The adoption of the term 'PA' in these studies is supported by Lorandos and Bernet (2020, p. 548). They determined that this label is the most frequently used in professional writing and everyday usage. They found that PA is 25% more frequent than the term 'PA syndrome' in common usage and is cited over 50% more often in professional writings (Lorandos & Bernet, 2020, p. 548). According to a search on Google, the phrase 'Parental Alienation' or 'PA' has become the most used phrase to describe this phenomenon (Lorandos & Bernet, 2020, p. 548).

The term 'adult survivor' signifies that the individual has endured and overcome adverse situations related to parental alienation during their formative years. This term suggests that they have navigated the challenges and impacts of SPA as they transitioned into adulthood. The inclusion of 'severe' emphasises the intensity and extent of the PA experienced by the individual. It acknowledges that the degree of alienation they encountered was profound, leading to significant and lasting effects on their well-being and relationships. Regarding the use of this term, it has been chosen to highlight the specific focus on individuals who have encountered severe levels of parental alienation during their upbringing. By utilising this term, the research aims to shed light on the unique perspectives and experiences of individuals who have faced such intense circumstances.

On the other hand, 'MHPs' refers to a diverse group of practitioners who work in the mental health field. This encompasses professionals from various backgrounds, including clinical psychotherapists, psychologists, psychiatrists, and counsellors. The term acknowledges the breadth of expertise and training in mental health. It recognises that MHPs are crucial in providing therapeutic support to individuals affected by SPA. Recognising the diversity within the group of MHPs is important as it acknowledges that different practitioners may approach and engage with adult survivors in distinct ways. The diverse backgrounds and therapeutic orientations of MHPs can contribute to various perspectives, practices, and experiences when working with adult survivors. Please note that this study refers to adult survivors of SPA as 'survivors' from this point unless distinguishing between child and adult survivors in the same sentence. 'Adult survivors' will retain their complete terminology in titles and direct quotations throughout the thesis.

Three Types of Pathogenic/Alienating Parents

Terminology concerning the adult actors in PA situations is limited by dualistic language and descriptors that can oversimplify the individual parents' roles, actions, and intentions. This narrow terminology fails to capture the complexity and nuances of their involvement in these situations. For example, the International Support Network of Alienated Families (ISNAF, 2021) uses the following terms to describe the adult actors in PA: An "Alienating Parent" refers to a parent who consciously or unconsciously causes a child to become alienated from the other parent. On the other hand, an "Alienated Parent" denotes a parent who has been unjustifiably and detrimentally alienated from their child due to interference, undermining, damage, or disruption in their relationship (ISNAF, 2021).

Three types of parents undertake to alienate their children from the other parent: naïve, active, and obsessive (Darnall,1998).

Naïve alienators acknowledge the value of the children's relationship with their other parent but occasionally say or act to alienate them. Sometimes, this is also performed unconsciously (Darnall, 1998).

Active alienators know better than to select this behaviour. However, when the triggers for internal dysregulation occur, they will often have a short-term loss of judgement and control (Darnall, 1998).

Obsessed alienators have a dedicated cause to destroy the other parent as they see them as betraying and abusing them and the shared child

(Darnall, 1998). They rationalise their behaviours by telling themselves that the child or themselves are being victimised and betrayed. Mental illness and personality disorders affect the obsessed parents' illogical thinking (Darnall, 1998). APs may also be described as obsessive alienators who persistently and frequently engage in many alienating behaviours with no willingness or ability to modify or correct these tactics (Lorandos & Bernet, 2020). "Obsessed alienators seem determined to destroy the child's relationship with the target parent" (Lorandos & Bernet, 2020, p. 551).

Personality disorders among APs encompass enduring and rigid patterns of inner thoughts and actions that deviate notably from societal norms (Baker, 2007). These patterns typically manifest during adolescence or early adulthood and have a lasting impact (Baker, 2007). Personality disorders encompass a broad range of maladaptive traits involving perception, emotional management, anxiety, and impulse control (Baker, 2007). They are prevalent mental disorders and often coexist with other conditions, such as substance use disorders, mood disorders, and anxiety disorders (American Psychiatric Association, 2013). Based on the descriptions of APs in Baker's (2007) research, many of them are considered as having Type B, Dramatic Personality Disorders. These disorders encompass antisocial, narcissistic, borderline, or histrionic traits (Baker, 2007). Individuals with these disorders often exhibit intense and unstable emotions, distorted self-perceptions, and impulsive behaviours (American Psychiatric Association, 2013).

The research will use the terms alienating parent and targeted parent as they focus on alienation's primary behaviour. However, the terms are used with caution, and the term SPA was explored in the extended literature review to avoid reductionism and dualistic constructions of a complex phenomenon. All the terms do not sufficiently indicate harmful interpersonal power dynamics or the impact of other actors and factors. Further, the research uses the term SPA as explained by Darnall (1998) and Lorandos & Bernet (2020), acknowledging the limitation of overly focusing on responding to an individual in strict adherence to levels that are not necessarily helpful to that individual.

Symptom Levels of PA- Mild, Moderate and Severe in Children

PA is commonly examined in relation to the varying degrees of severity experienced by the child involved. According to Gardner (1998), the dynamics of PA manifest in three distinct levels of symptoms: mild, moderate, and severe. Each level requires a significantly different approach to address PA's effects on the child (Gardner, 1998).

Mild Parental Alienation

The mild type of PA behaviour is considered to have some degree of parental programming aimed against the TP; however, visits are not detrimentally affected, and the child can manage the transition to be around the alienated TP without too much stress (Baker, 2007). A mild level of PA is also identified when the child resisting contact with the TP starts to enjoy parenting time and relinquishes the resistance they were displaying at the start of the visit (Lorandos & Bernet, 2020, p. 550).

Moderate Parental Alienation

According to Baker (2007), the moderate type of PA is more fearsome, the children are more unruly and insolent, and the campaign of abuse may be almost constant. A moderate level of PA is identified when the child exhibits strong resistance to the suggestion of contact with their TP and is constantly opposed during parenting time visits, apart from the few moments of encouraging connection between the child and AP (Lorandos & Bernet, 2020, p. 550). A further example of moderate PAS would be characterised as the child being exposed to a considerable level of parental programming from the AP. This programming creates a substantial internal battle for the child when visiting a TP (Baker, 2007, p. 22). In these cases, the child may have trouble adjusting to the dynamics of the visit with the TP. Still, their relationship is reasonably strong, and eventually, they settle and adapt to the visit (Baker, 2007)

For a child experiencing SPA, their behaviours are usually due to the AP's obsessional goal to destroy the relationship between the TP and the child (Lorandos et al., 2013). When it comes time for the children to be with the TP, the children can display behaviours that can be highly oppositional, especially if the AP encourages them to act this way toward the TP (Lorandos et al., 2013). In the case of severely alienated children and their TPs, this interference can cause their relationship to be destroyed entirely (Baker, 2007).

Severe Parental Alienation

In cases experiencing severe levels of SPA, children are adamant in their hatred of the alienated TP, often refusing visits with them and threatening to run away if a visit is proposed (Baker, 2007). Children experiencing severe levels of PA often have an unhealthy, enmeshed alliance with the AP, sharing paranoid fantasies about the TP to the point where the child's relationship with the TP is destroyed (Baker, 2007). Friends and family may also notice that the child and AP may have an unhealthy alliance (Baker, 2007). The definition of severe parental alienation (SPA), according to Lorandos et al. (2013), involves children who persistently and adamantly refuse all contact with the TP to the extent that they may even run away or hide to avoid spending time with them. Within the SPA context, visitation may be impossible due to the children being incredibly hostile to the point where the children may become physically violent toward the supposedly hated parent (Baker, 2007).

Other ways of acting out may be present, designed to cause formidable grief to the parent visited by the alienated child (Baker, 2007). These levels can manifest in behaviours such as running away and hiding to avoid seeing the alienated parent and remaining defiant and oppositional if they are made to spend parenting time with them (Baker, 2007). In addition, some severely alienated children exhibit behaviours such as persisting in not seeing the alienated parent and stating that they do not want to partake in a relationship with them (Lorandos & Bernet, 2020, p. 550). "In many cases, the children's hostility has reached paranoid levels, that is, delusions of persecution and fears that they will be murdered in situations where there is absolutely no evidence that such will be the case" (Gardner, 2008, p. 2).

Research Issue

Over 3.8 million children in the United States of America are reported to be moderately to severely alienated from one of their parents (Harman et al., 2019). Researchers estimate that approximately 20 million children in the United States of America are already the victims of mild, moderate, and severe parental alienation (Opperman, 2004). As of May 2023, no comparative studies are available reporting the precise number of survivors of SPA in Australia.

Use of Older References

To address the use of the Researcher using older references in these studies, it is important to note that researchers have primarily focused on children affected by PA rather than adult survivors. This is why earlier research on survivors of PA and SPA has been relied upon. To verify this, the Researcher contacted an expert in SPA research who confirmed that no recent studies on survivors of PA had been published in the past two years. The extended use of referencing Baker's research is primarily due to her prominent role as a leading researcher in the field of survivors of PA. However, it is crucial to recognise that Baker's research has certain limitations and does not explicitly target adults affected by SPA.

Survivors of SPA are not recognised as having complex trauma stemming from child maltreatment. A lack of recognition of survivors may be due to the paucity of research. Results from both cohorts in these studies reported a dearth of MHPs taught to recognise or identify SPA. A secondary complication within this phenomenon is that the MHPs who treat this cohort may find themselves at a loss as to how to treat the complex trauma experienced by the adult survivor. In addition, practitioners may also be exposed to vicarious, social-emotional, and neurobiological trauma (Garber, 2004).

Available research literature relating to the therapeutic needs of survivors appears limited. One resource book briefly addressing clinical considerations as a guide when working with survivors of mild PA, not SPA, is "Adult Children of Parental Alienation Syndrome: Breaking the Ties that Bind" (Baker, 2007). In addition, other self-help books are available for adult children of divorce in the grey literature category; however, the information given does not extend to contents pertaining to MHPs or suggest which therapeutic approaches would be preferable for practitioners to undertake with survivors.

A second book that provides a methodology for assessing and providing intervention strategies for children experiencing PA was compiled by Haines et al., 2020. These strategies use a therapeutic approach based on psychological theory and methods. Psychological intervention for children within the PA framework is driven by reunification with their TP while helping them cope with and resolve any psychological distress they may be experiencing due to family dysfunction (Haines et al., 2020).

Research suggests that the relationships that children experience cause them to interact in particular ways, establishing a blueprint for all their subsequent relationships (Critchfield & Benjamin, 2008). This finding is a serious issue because adults who have grown up with experiences of child abuse and maltreatment have lived a life with inadequate secure attachment, encouragement, guidance, and nurturance from primary caregivers, leaving them with substantial deficits in which to enter life as an adult (Ellis et al., 2019, p. 167). This concept is explained further in 'Key Concepts: Attachment and Abandonment'.

Many professionals argue that PA and the associated behaviours accompanying this phenomenon and its impact on children are classified as child maltreatment and abuse. According to Saini et al. (2019, p. 107), "Child abuse is a major public health concern and a strong predictor of adult psychopathology". Research shows that few MHPs receive the supervision and training required within trauma psychology and traumatic stress studies (Cook et al., 2011). The Diagnostics and Statistics Manual-5 defines child abuse as "non-accidental verbal or symbolic acts by a child's parent or caregiver that result or have a reasonable potential to result in significant psychological harm to the child" (American Psychiatric Association, 2013, p. 719).

Early research suggests that survivors are prone to approximately twice the risk of experiencing other forms of abuse, such as sexual harassment and rape (Herman, 1992, p. 387). In addition, survivors identify six key areas resulting from multiple traumas associated with parental alienation syndrome (PAS), affecting their functioning (Baker, 2007, p. 320). These areas are identified as "low self-esteem, lack of trust in themselves and others, depression, drug and alcohol problems, alienation from their children, and [parental] divorce" (Baker, 2007, p. 320).

Individuals who have undergone severe alienation and child abuse as survivors of SPA may exhibit various symptoms. Some researchers describe these symptoms as behavioural impairments, such as displaying extreme hostility, defiance, withdrawal, and disobedience; emotional impairments, including openly expressing contempt and a lack of genuine love, appreciation, or affection; and cognitive impairments (Gardner, 1998; Kelly, 2010). Symptoms include trivial complaints about the rejected parent, echoing the AP and claiming the words to be their own. Adults exposed to multiple traumas during childhood "develop significant and behavioural health difficulties" (Courtois & Ford, 2009; Kilpatrick et al., 2003). Traumatic exposure during childhood is identified as a risk factor for several major mental disorders, including substance abuse/dependence, depression, post-traumatic stress disorder (PTSD) and associated anxiety disorders (Green et al., 2010; McLaughlin et al., 2010), personality and developmental disorders and disturbances and dissociative disorders (Cook et al., 2011). For example, adverse physical effects are the number one cause of death in adults who have experienced complex trauma as children (Felitti et al., 1998). These are cancer, ischemic heart disease, chronic lung disease, liver disease, skeletal fractures, and poor self-related health (Felitti et al., 1998). Adverse psychological effects can include anxiety disorders, depression, low self-esteem, guilt, lack of trust (Baker, 2007), cognitive dissonance, and false memories (Haines et al., 2020). This list is not exhaustive; adverse effects on survivors are investigated in the following chapters.

It is essential to investigate further the impact of SPA on survivors, which treatments they are engaging in, and which are helping. To date, the phenomenon of SPA has been continually noted regarding children of prolonged, high-conflict custody and visitation disputes, yet existing literature on what life is like after the child exposed to SPA develops into an adult is sparse. Previous literature on the impacts of PA has been universally observed and described as having detrimental psychological effects (Verrocchio et al., 2016). Impacts include severe short-term consequences on the child victims and long-term sequelae for survivors of PA (Verrocchio et al., 2016). The more often a child is exposed to neglect or abuse, the worse the outcome for survivors may be, which negatively impacts the child's neurobiological development, relational skills, risk-taking behaviours, and psychological and physical health (Peterson et al., 2014).

Additionally, trauma is correlated with negative health behaviours such as excessive consumption of alcohol, smoking, lesser social and work-related functioning ability, and an overall lower quality of life (Kessler, 2000). Due to this scarcity of information about therapeutic treatment for survivors, the research will draw upon 'related parallel trauma areas' listed as another dimension of PA in more depth in Chapter Two. Examples of co-occurring child maltreatment areas drawn upon will be child abduction, child kidnapping, child filicide, child sexual abuse (CSA), family and domestic violence, grief and loss, factitious disorder imposed on another, Stockholm syndrome, intergenerational cycles of trauma and violence, exploitation, and torture. These examples will be drawn from previous studies based on child maltreatment and abuse in childhood to give context as a contemporary source of the systematic nature of abuse.

The Researchers' positionality and motivation for these studies derive from personal experience as an adult survivor of SPA and Abduction (SPAA) and professional practice as a clinical psychotherapist who treats other survivors, APs, and TPs. Chapter Four, titled Methodology, provides comprehensive information on how the Researcher conducted the study to mitigate bias and ensure accurate results. It outlines the specific approaches and techniques employed to address potential biases throughout the research process. The term "Severe Parental Alienation and Abduction as a Child" (SPAA) refers to a complex situation where a child has experienced both SPA and abduction during their upbringing. "Abduction as a child" refers to the act of unlawfully taking or retaining a child without the consent of a custodial parent or legal guardian, often resulting in the child being removed from their familiar environment, disrupted from established relationships, and subjected to emotional distress and potential harm (Hickey & Nedim, 2020). When these two experiences are combined under the term SPAA, it signifies that the child has not only endured SPA but has also been subjected to the traumatic experience of being abducted, further exacerbating the complexity and impact on the child's well-being.

The Researcher designed these studies due to noticing a lack of education and understanding regarding SPA in her own mental health community. Therefore, results from this research will contribute to knowledge for other researchers to build upon while helping to combat this widespread community problem. The Researcher also observes that MHPs struggle to understand PA, SPA and SPAA among survivors due to a lack of specialist PA training. This lack of training adversely affects the client and their MHPs, as reported in Volume Two, Chapters Five and Six. This knowledge gap has adverse implications for clients and their MHPs and holds critical importance in court proceedings concerning divorce and cases of PA and SPA in Australia. With the rise in divorce rates during the early 1970s, studies on divorce emerged, and mental health professionals began presenting instances of PA to the Family Court.

The Adverse Childhood Experiences Study

These studies' findings shed light on the long-lasting effects such adverse experiences can have on individuals, reinforcing the importance of understanding the impact of childhood experiences on overall well-being. Speaking to this issue, the Adverse Childhood Experiences Study (ACES), conducted by Kaiser Permanente Health Maintenance Organisation and the Centers for Disease Control and Prevention, investigated this subject between 1996 and 1997 (Centers for Disease Control and Prevention, 2020).

The ACE Study is the leading ongoing investigation between childhood maltreatment and adult health from data collected from over 17,000 participants. Two waves of data collection surveyed people in Southern California who participated in physical exams. The residents filled out confidential surveys pertaining to their childhood experiences, current health status, and associated behaviours (Centers for Disease Control and Prevention, 2020). The ACE Study discovered how developmental risk factors for disease are related to well-being during a lifetime (Centers for Disease Control and Prevention, 2020). In addition, the "Family Health History and Health Appraisal" questionnaires collated data on child abuse and neglect, household challenges such as divorce and separation, and other relevant socio-behavioural factors (Centers for Disease Control and Prevention, 2020).

The study reports that "negative experiences in childhood and the teenage years may put children at risk for chronic health problems, mental illness, and substance use in adulthood" (Centers for Disease

Control and Prevention, 2020, p. 1). The lasting effects on adults who have experienced ACEs include suicide, lower job opportunities, and a wide range of chronic diseases, including heart disease, cancer, and diabetes (Centers for Disease Control and Prevention, 2020). Sexually transmitted diseases, pregnancy complications, foetal death, maternal and child health problems, risk of injury and sex trafficking are potential consequences (Centers for Disease Control and Prevention, 2020).

Furthermore, children exposed to toxic stress may have difficulty forming stable, healthy relationships as adults and struggle with finances, depression, and job unpredictability (Centers for Disease Control and Prevention, 2020). An important fact to consider regarding the ACES is that it was conducted over 20 years ago with people born from the 1930s to the 1950s, and divorce was rare and heavily stigmatised.

The ACES measures ten different types of childhood trauma. The first five are listed as personal- "physical abuse, verbal abuse, sexual abuse, physical neglect, and emotional neglect. Five are related to other family members: a parent who's an alcoholic, a mother who's a victim of domestic violence, a family member in jail, a family member diagnosed with a mental illness, and experiencing the divorce of parents" (ACES Too High News, 2020, p. 1). For every trauma a person identifies with, they receive a score of one point. Note: the above web reference 'ACES Too High' was used as the link to the same information previously available on the Centre for Disease Control website, which has not been connected for a few months.

ACE Study Scores 4-10

The study findings showed that a significant majority, precisely 87% of participants, scored higher than one point among the two-thirds of individuals who participated. A noteworthy observation was that an ACE score exceeding 4 indicates a greater level of trauma and severity, which practitioners should note. Such a score corresponds to a significantly elevated probability of developing chronic pulmonary lung disease by 390%. Additionally, there is a heightened probability of developing hepatitis at 240%, experiencing depression at a 460% higher risk, and attempting suicide with a concerning 1,220% likelihood (ACES Too High News, 2020). See Appendix Two ACE Study Questions. Furthermore, these studies emphasise the significance of incorporating the concept of ACEs and recognising the presence of CITs when providing therapeutic support to survivors.

Key Concepts: Attachment and Abandonment

Key concepts featured in the research pertaining to survivors will include attachment, abandonment, complex trauma, lack of recognition and the harm done to survivors. For the practitioners, key concepts will be that SPA is not recognised as complex trauma due to a lack of education and professional training.

Attachment

Attachment theory explains that the quality of early parent-child interactions leads to a child's ability to regulate emotions, integrate a sense of self, and foster the capacity for secure relationships in later life (Bowlby, 1982). Attachment also refers to the condition and calibre of an individual's emotional connection with a significant other (Bowlby, 1980). In parent-child relationships, a healthy attachment necessitates warmth, empathy, and consistent engagement to facilitate the child's optimal development (Bowlby, 1988). Attachment behaviour encompasses any actions undertaken to establish and maintain proximity with another person who is perceived as more adept at navigating the world (Bowlby, 1988). For example, alienated children commonly exhibit insecure attachment toward the AP due to the latter's inclination to prioritise their own needs over fostering a consistently warm and empathically engaged relationship with the child (Haines et al., 2020).

However, when PA is involved, one of the child's attachment figures, the TP, will be erased from their lives (Haines et al., 2020). This will result in the child having no choice but to attach to the AP and becoming forced to make them the primary attachment figure (Haines et al., 2020). Consequently, the child will exhibit attachment behaviours due to a fear of losing another attachment figure (Haines et al., 2020). Practitioners who work with children of PA may interpret this behaviour as "fear of the targeted parent" and may miss the parent-child interactions and attachment styles playing out in the session (Haines et al., 2020). In addition, alienated children often show signs of insecure attachment toward the AP due to the AP prioritising their needs over creating an ongoing, warm, empathic relationship with their child (Haines et al., 2020).

As MHPs seek to address the impacts of childhood trauma, such as SPA, it is important to examine various factors that may have contributed to the development of attachment styles. Attachment styles can often be intergenerational, so exploring the AP and TPs attachment styles is prudent (Haines et al., 2020). In addition to attachment styles, MHPs will also need to explore the potential impacts of abandonment, which has been documented as a prevalent issue among survivors of childhood trauma. For instance, in Baker's (2007) study, two adult children shared their experiences of abandonment, as explained in the following section.

Abandonment

The two adult children in Baker's (2007) study explained their stories of abandonment and how they felt it had stemmed from PA. The first "adult child" explained, "I had intense abandonment issues and fears of intimacy. I doubted my mother's love and felt rejected by my biological father, believing he despised me" (Baker, 2007, p. 246). The second "adult child" explained, "As a result of a significant emotional experience during my youth, I struggle with finding stability. With 12 years in Alcoholics Anonymous, I am convinced that I have grappled with the effects of abandonment and severe emotional and mental disorders" (Baker, 2007, p. 310).

Baker (2007) reports that APs use the threat of abandonment as fuel to convince children of PA that the TP has never loved them and sow seeds of doubt about the TP's parenting skills and commitment to the relationship with the child. Along with the threat of abandonment, these children may have also been threatened with mutilation or, ultimately, death. The detrimental consequences arising from complex trauma resulting from ongoing threats can manifest as distressing and overt expressions of emotional abuse, characterised by repetitive and cumulative occurrences within a specific relationship over an extended period (Courtois, 2004, p. 412).

Previous research reports that PA and its associated complex trauma may negatively impact children and adolescent PA survivors' mental health through expressions of guilt, depressed mood, low self-esteem, lack of self-confidence, and distress and frustration. This negative impact can lead to substance abuse, delinquent behaviour, separation anxiety, suicidal ideation, suicide attempts, sleep and eating disorders, educational difficulties, hypochondria, psychosomatic illness, encopresis, enuresis, and fears and phobias (Sher, 2017), especially when there is a family breakdown leading to divorce.

Children's lives are intrinsically linked to their families, caregivers, and parents. When a divorce occurs, the transitioning of the family affects children directly and indirectly. Multiple aspects of the child's life can be impacted by divorce, particularly when the changes become challenging and overwhelming. Key impact themes that children of divorce may face include changes in physical movements, financial circumstances, changes in their roles and social life, changes in education and career development and experiencing complex emotional loss states (Das, 2016). Garber (2004) reports that the children of highly opposed caregivers are among those most in need of psychotherapeutic assistance and are also the most difficult to assist in the psychotherapeutic process.

Behavioural Impairments of Severely Alienated Children

Psychologist and author Dr Richard Warshak (2013) describes the behavioural impairments of severely alienated children that adult survivors may have experienced during childhood. Warshak (2013) explains that children who have been severely alienated will treat the TP with extreme hostility, defiance, disobedience, and withdrawal. They may resist and reject contact, threaten and perpetrate violence and vandalise and steal property. One example from Warshak's (2013) experience with a young, severely alienated child in Court reports, "A boy told the custody evaluator that he would like to give his father a hard kick between the legs, kill him in his sleep, and have him die a horrible death". This level of venom is characteristic of children at the severe end of the PA continuum (Warshak, 2013).

Behavioural impairments experienced by children of SPA report that these children often behave well among other adults, apart from the TP and anyone who associates with them. By contrast, children who are physically abused fear their abuser and act respectfully, compliant, and obsequiously to avoid angering their parent, as opposed to children of SPA who do not openly disrespect or defy the alienating, abusive parent. Physically abused children will also want to stay with their parent, and if there is a separation, they will want to return to them (Warshak, 2013).

Critical thinking regarding their parents is not evidenced in children referred to as irrationally or severely alienated. Instead, the child of SPA will demonstrate unwavering, involuntary support of the APs position whenever the parents disagree (Warshak, 2013). Some children of SPA may go as far as to testify in Court against their TP, lobby on the APs' behalf during litigation, or speak to the judge in Court on behalf of their AP. Warshak (2013 p.2) explains the most pernicious sign of unreasonable alienation as being what he calls "hatred by association." This term describes the spread of hatred by the child of SPA toward anyone associated with the TP, as well as objects, therapists, extended family, and pets.

Children of SPA also learn to "curry favour" with the AP by echoing the parents' complaining words about the TP (Warshak, 2013). They learn quickly that the AP can become displeased if they show affection or connection to the TP. They may also refer to the TP by their first name or a name of derision, apart from mum or dad (Warshak, 2013). Although many onlookers will see clearly that the child has been strongly influenced against the TP by the AP, the child of SPA will never agree to such an influence. Often, the child will blame the TP and relatives for provoking the hatred in them while only providing vague reasons for rejecting their other parent (Baker, 2007). When these children grow into survivors, and because they have been exposed to multiple traumas during childhood, they will "develop significant behavioural and health difficulties" (Courtois & Ford, 2009; Kilpatrick et al., 2003).

New Specific Phobia-Severe Parental Alienation and Abduction Anxiety Variant

Further investigation is needed to develop targeted interventions for survivors of severe parental alienation and abduction (SPAA) who may also have experienced factitious disorder imposed on another (FDIOA) or shared delusional disorder (SDD) during childhood. Understanding the nuanced symptoms associated with these complex interpersonal traumas is essential for effective intervention strategies.

The Researcher posits that children who have experienced both SPAA and FDIOA are more likely to develop the potential new anxiety variant identified in this research. The previous multiple trauma description was evidenced in 75% of the survivor participants who had experienced SPA, abduction, and potential FDIOA by their APs. Within this survivor group data, the Researcher uncovered a new specific phobia, namely the "Specific Phobia-Severe Parental Alienation and Abduction Anxiety Variant" (Price-Tobler, 2023).

This variant developed because 30% of the survivors in these studies did not agree with Warshak's (2013) description regarding the behaviour of young children and adolescents toward their TPs, as previously mentioned. Instead, the study participants who experienced the CIT involving SPAA under the age of eight reported anxiety and phobic-type symptoms that had not been documented as far as the Researcher knew. Consequently, as these symptoms differed from the descriptions regarding children experiencing SPA symptoms in earlier research, the Researcher documented and investigated these new SPAA symptoms, which developed into a new sub-variant of SPA. Please refer to Key Theme Four, namely 'Potential New Discovery Found Due to Being a Lived Experience Researcher' for more information.

Previous research has reported that experiencing parental divorce as a child is a predictor of adverse outcomes when they become adults. Furthermore, there is a dearth of information regarding SPA studies on the lifelong effects on survivors. However, Das (2016, p. 12) refers to the work of Duran-Aydintug (1997) and Amato and Sobolewski (2001) and informs that "adult children of divorce show lower scores on measures of psychological, social, and marital well-being as compared to other adults". Studies suggest reduced physical health, increased behavioural problems, lower financial status, and fewer educational opportunities. Further studies also indicate that adult children of divorce may experience elevated levels of interpersonal and emotional problems and more difficult parent-child relationships (Das, 2016).

Researchers report that individuals who grow up perceiving exposure to PA from childhood maltreatment may experience significant adverse effects relating to their 'health-related quality of life' (HRQol) (Verrocchio et al., 2019, p. 2). Survivors of PA are also likely to experience long-lasting consequences, including depressive symptoms that can affect their daily lives well into adulthood (Verrocchio et al., 2019). Numerous adverse outcomes can last throughout adulthood, such as chronic health, substance abuse, mental illness, educational impacts, and lack of job opportunities (Centers for Disease Control and Prevention, 2020). Long-term effects on survivors of PA include depression, low self-esteem, lack of trust, drug and alcohol abuse, and divorce. Survivors may also alienate themselves from their children to avoid further rejection and a lack of belonging or choose not to have children (Sher, 2017). They may also experience suicidality, resentment and bitterness over time lost with their alienated parent (Sher, 2017). Baker's (2007) research mirrored the previous results from Verrocchio et al. (2019), reporting that the long-term effects of PA on adult children manifest in depression, divorce, substance abuse, trust issues in themselves and others, and alienation from their offspring.

Furthermore, Baker (2007, p.149) highlighted that the negative long-term consequences of parental alienation on survivors were further exacerbated by the harmful practice of terrorising children, which involves "singling them out for criticism and punishment". Baker (2007) explains that APs who choose this form of emotional abuse will often ridicule the child for showing normal emotions and have expectations of the child far beyond their capability. One example by adult survivor "Aurora" whose alienating mother had succeeded in removing all traces of her targeted father, describes her experience in the following extract;

> It felt like death with no funeral for my father, and the pain has gone on for fifty-two years. I was closest to my father when I was young, and I lived with him until age four when my mother and stepfather abducted me and started the severe PA toward my father. Recovery for me is not something I think will happen. I just have to live with what they did.

The research further acknowledges that individuals from diverse backgrounds can be susceptible to complex trauma. For example, a war veteran and a child being abused at home may show signs of PTSD despite their vastly different traumas. Shifts in psychiatry and traumatology recognise that traditional mental health diagnoses, such as PTSD, do not effectively capture the effects of prolonged and multiple categories of victimisation (Briere & Spinazzola, 2005; Herman J, 1992).

The DSM-5 and SPA

Several studies have produced reports on the symptoms and deficits experienced by survivors. However, there is still insufficient data from qualitative studies that compare differences in therapeutic experiences for this cohort and the practitioners who work with them. Consequently, survivors of PA may seek therapy from MHPs to help them understand and move through this healing process. Unfortunately, many MHPs are unaware of the unique phenomena of PA, nor are they trained to work with survivors of PA or SPA and the varying adverse outcomes predicted for their lives.

MHPs look toward the Diagnostic and Statistical Manual of Mental Disorders-5 (DSM-5) for diagnosis and treatment options. The DSM-5 manual endorses a common language and basic measures that MHPs use to classify mental disorders. However, the term PA is not in the DSM-5. Currently, the closest definition to PA in the DSM-5 is the term "child affected by parental relationship distress (CAPRD)", which was added to the most recent edition of the DSM-5 (Harman, 2016, p.2). However, the authors of the DSM-5 clarify that "child affected by parental relationship distress" (CAPRD) does include many of the recognised PA effects and behaviours (Harman, 2016, p.2). Due to the scarcity of information on therapeutic treatment for survivors, the research will draw upon related parallel trauma areas often listed as another dimension of PA or complex intersecting traumas (CITs) from previous studies. These studies are based on child maltreatment and abuse in childhood to give context as a contemporary source of the systematic nature of abuse in more depth in Chapter Three, 'An Extended Literature Review'.

The research will explore the therapeutic relationship and understanding of the respective experiences of MHPs who work with survivors. For example, the associated symptoms experienced by survivors may prompt them to seek help from MHPs, who, in turn, may find themselves experiencing a lack of knowledge and understanding of the effects of SPA and facing adverse effects of vicarious trauma while listening to SPA recounts. The concept of vicarious traumatisation refers to the continuing transformative impact experienced by therapists due to their empathetic involvement with clients who have been traumatised (McCann & Pearlman, 1990).

The Impact of PA on MHPs

Due to a dearth of research on the impact on MHPs who work with survivors, the closest comparison study results were on MHPs working with children experiencing PAS. This study reported that "the impact of working with such a complex phenomenon has emotional effects like self-doubt, disappointment, and anxiety, and in some cases, this resulted in an active decision on the part of the psychologist not to work with forensic cases anymore" (Viljoen & van Rensburg, 2014, p. 253). Results from the interviews with MHPs who work with survivors are presented in Volume Two.

Research indicates that intervening in PA cases involving children can be therapeutically challenging. However, the tailored evidence-based intervention programs currently emerging in the literature aim to protect children from further harm within the design of their structure and processes (Haines et al., 2020). Existing literature reports that current intervention programs are based on available PA research findings and behavioural change standards, with all the programs having carefully designed protocols to assist practitioners in intervening in mild to severe cases of PA, even though there are some differences between the programs (Haines et al., 2020).

Evidence currently developing from these programs indicates an improved degree of psychological well-being within the child, combined with enhanced critical thinking skills and reduced levels of distorted thinking commonly seen in children of alienation (Haines et al., 2020). However, critics opposing this evidence argue that the research has been limited due to the reliance on qualitative data analysis with no information sourced that matches cases together or accesses information from a control group (Haines et al., 2020). In addition, no evidence-based programs are available for survivors to help them recover.

Baker's (2007) study reports that risk factors for PAS are similar to symptoms of other maltreatment, namely sexual abuse, emotional abuse, physical abuse, poor impulse control, alcoholism, and personality disorders. Therefore, these must all be considered as they could be relevant to the adult survivor's treatment (Baker, 2007). Baker (2007) also reported that the frequency of physical and sexual abuse was higher for the adult children of PAS than the overall population. Furthermore, MHPs who work with survivors of PA need to know how to treat a disorder that involves the attachment system (Childress, 2015). Finally, treatment for survivors requires a thorough knowledge of both the patterns and manifestations of PA (Baker, 2007, p. 361), as survivor indicators can be complex and hidden by a disguised presentation (Gelinas, 1983). The Researcher has incorporated Gelinas' (1983) reference because her work on incest is a related parallel trauma to PA, providing valuable insights into the concept of 'disguised presentation'. Research reports that clients who come into therapy don't often realise that what they have experienced during their childhood does have a name, even though PA is a relatively new phenomenon that has not seeped into mainstream consciousness yet (Baker, 2007). Consequently, an adult survivor may go through a 'realisation' stage where they discover that one of their parents had turned them against the other for their own need to control, seek revenge, and gain emotional satisfaction at the expense of the child (Baker, 2007).

Due to the risk factors for PA being similar to other types of abuse, such as personality disorders, low impulse control, family tension and alcoholism, practitioners must draw upon current literature to work with this special population (Baker, 2007). However, earlier studies indicate that when survivors present with complex trauma symptoms during the realisation stage, it is difficult for practitioners to identify the diverse range of symptoms and determine the most suitable treatments. This lack of recognition highlights the need for further research and understanding in this area, as it is currently vastly understudied.

MHPs Training

Recent public awareness campaigns promoting better mental health for community members have increased recognition of available help for trauma survivors. This increased awareness highlights the need for MHPs to undergo specialised training in trauma counselling to deliver adequate treatment. As this research data on survivors and their specialised treatment needs continue to develop, preparing for the expanding population requiring specialised care is crucial. Additionally, these studies report that further information is needed regarding MHPs' current therapeutic practice patterns, the implementation of clinical training programs, and the monitoring of vicarious trauma on practitioners. Chapter Six reports on preliminary findings and effective treatment suggestions to better understand this burgeoning topic. Furthermore, it is important to acknowledge the historical context of psychiatric treatment options for children affected by Parental Alienation Syndrome, as outlined in the following topic.

Aims of the Study

The overarching research question driving this study revolves around the perspectives of survivors of SPA and the MHPs who work with them therapeutically by addressing the following aims:

Main Question

1. What are the perspectives of adult survivors of SPA and the MHPs who work with them to address the symptoms of SPA during therapy?

Sub Questions

1a. What are the perspectives of adult survivors of SPA regarding their consultations with MHPs during and or after therapy to treat symptoms pertaining to SPA?

1b. What are the perspectives of MHPs who work with adult survivors of SPA pertaining to their symptomology?

The aims of these studies were twofold. The first aim was to gain a deeper understanding of the lived experiences and perspectives of individuals who identify as survivors of SPA and have undergone traditional therapeutic treatments. By examining their personal narratives, the research sought to uncover the survivor's unique insights into the methods and treatments that proved helpful in their journey towards healing and recovery. This exploration aimed to demystify the often-under-researched phenomenon of survivors, shedding light on their experiences with MHPs and offering valuable recommendations for improving therapeutic practices. The term "therapeutic practice" is crucial to establish as an aspect of the research because it focuses on the methods, approaches, and interventions employed by MHPs when working with survivors of SPA. By examining therapeutic practices, the research aims to gain insights into the strategies, techniques, therapies, and modalities MHPs use to address survivors' unique needs and challenges. Understanding therapeutic practice allows for exploring the effectiveness, limitations, and potential areas of improvement in the therapeutic interventions provided to survivors. It provides an opportunity to evaluate the relevance and applicability of different approaches and identify best practices that may lead to better outcomes for this population.

The second aim of the research focused on examining the perspectives, practices, and experiences of MHPs working directly with survivors of SPA. By engaging with these professionals, the study aimed to comprehensively understand the current therapeutic approaches utilised in the PA field. This involved investigating the treatments employed by MHPs, identifying what they perceive as helpful or unhelpful practices, and exploring their training backgrounds. The research aimed to uncover valuable insights and recommendations from MHPs, allowing for the development of therapeutic interventions for survivors of SPA. By exploring the survivor perspectives and the experiences of MHPs, these studies aimed to contribute to the professional knowledge base surrounding SPA, ultimately leading to improved therapeutic approaches that better address survivors' complex needs and experiences.

The study was also designed to address the issue of no recommendations for best practices for MHPs who work with this vulnerable population. Previous research reports that MHPs are unclear as to which therapeutic technique, or combination, is the best practice to support this unique population. For example, Fidler and Bala (2010) explain that "counselling or psychotherapy tend to be suitable in mild to moderate cases, but not in extreme cases" (Fidler & Bala, 2010, p. 24). Many mental health and legal professionals who work with divorcing families have recognised PA as a phenomenon (Verrocchio et al., 2019). As a result, thousands of psychiatrists, psychologists, social workers, and family counsellors are also treating PA (Verrocchio et al., 2019).

Chapter Two

Related Parallel Trauma

The dearth of information available on adult survivors of SPA justifies the inclusion of Chapter Two in this research. Given the limited existing knowledge in this specific area, the Researcher needed to draw from related parallel trauma areas to gather insights. By examining related parallel trauma areas and co-occurring maltreatment themes, Chapter Two establishes a contextual framework highlighting the systematic nature of abuse, as discussed in Chapter One.

Through this research, it is hypothesised that chronic exposure to emotional abuse and the disruption of the child's attachment to the TP can lead to profound psychological consequences. Additionally, the study examines the potential link between SPA and the development of mental health disorders. The Researcher theorises that the chronic invalidation, gaslighting, and manipulation experienced through PABs can disrupt the child's development of a cohesive and integrated sense of self, potentially contributing to the emergence of identity disorders.

This research aims to provide a nuanced understanding of the relationship between SPA and dissociation, identity disorders, and other psychological outcomes by exploring the specific mechanisms through which SPA impacts these factors. It seeks to shed light on the unique psychological challenges children and adults exposed to SPA face and inform interventions and support strategies to address these complex issues effectively.

This contextual information is crucial because survivors may have experienced various related parallel trauma areas and CITs that MHPs may not know. By considering these related themes, the research aims to develop a more comprehensive understanding of survivors' complex needs, which will inform appropriate interventions and support strategies to promote healing and recovery.

Furthermore, the chapter also addresses the need for MHPs to be aware of disguised trauma presentations. These disguised presentations are described as concealed or indirect manifestations of trauma, as discussed by Gelinas (1983). By familiarising MHPs with these disguised presentations, the research aims to enhance their ability to effectively identify and address trauma-related issues, even when the survivor may not be aware that this is what is happening to them.

The subsequent chapters build upon the foundation established in this chapter. They provide detailed reporting of the CITs identified through interviews conducted with survivors and MHPs who work with them. By presenting direct trauma examples, these chapters offer firsthand and contemporary insight into the direct impact on survivors, further contributing to understanding SPA and its consequences.

Suicide of a Targeted Parent Due to Alienation

MHPs working with survivors must be aware of related parallel trauma and associated CITs that may have or may still be impacting survivors' lives. One such dimension involves the suicide of a survivor's TP due to the alienation and strategies used against them by the AP. For example, a previous study of fifty-four self-referred TPs alienated from their children found that 23% of the participants who volunteered for the study had attempted suicide at some point due to the consequences of the alienation against them and the coping strategies they employed (Lee-Maturana et al., 2000, p.1). Some TPs reported that they had attempted suicide on more than one occasion. Other study participants reflected that their suffering had been too great, and they had considered suicide to resolve their suffering. Alarmingly, 44% of the participants had described how they were not coping well. Consequently, the researchers expressed an urgency for a better understanding of the TP and for mental health and legal practitioners to be watchful of the needs of TPs. Regarding survivors, MHPs need to consider that they may have had a parent attempt suicide but failed, or the parent may have completed suicide.

Child Abduction and Divorce in Australia

Another dimension of SPA and related parallel trauma is child family abduction, also known in Australia as parental child abduction (Hickey & Nedim, 2020). Parental child abduction is against Australian law and is listed as a criminal offence under the Family Law Act, providing there are orders in place or a Court proceeding involving the child (Hickey & Nedim, 2020). Parental child abduction usually occurs when two parents are engaged in a high-conflict custody dispute and are described as "when one parent takes, detains or conceals a child from the other parent, and it is not uncommon for other family members to help the abducting parent" (Hickey & Nedim, 2020, p. 1). New laws were created in 2018 to ensure that "these offences also extend to any persons acting on behalf of a person to whom the provisions apply, and it is also a crime to *attempt* to commit this type of offence» (Hickey & Nedim, 2020, p. 1). Carrying out this offence incurs a maximum sentence of three years in prison.

Parental Child Abduction Ring in Australia

In Australia, a criminal law article on child abuse and divorce reported that a parental child abduction ring operating in Queensland was available to hire for $1,500 to help disgruntled parents abduct their child to stop the other parent from having a visitation or gaining access to the child (Hickey & Nedim, 2020). Nine people were charged concerning the "sophisticated operation" of the ring. However, others involved in the operation, some who have not been to Court since this article was created, have been charged with child stealing, stalking and conspiracy to defeat justice (Hickey & Nedim, 2020, p. 1). In addition, one of the men who procured the parental child abduction ring services was sentenced to an 18-month good behaviour bond for payments made within a contract to have his child abducted.

Child Abduction and Divorce in America

The US Department of Justice reports that there are possibly more than 200,000 children who are currently victims of child family abduction each year (Office of Juvenile Justice and Delinquency Prevention, 2010). The fact sheet from The Center for The Study of Traumatic Stress cites that the US Department of Justice has reported even higher numbers for non-familial abductions, between 3,200-4,600 per year (University of the Health Sciences, 2021). No year date was mentioned.

Furthermore, a parent or family member takes the majority of children, and family abduction remains overloaded with myths and misconceptions. The effects on the missing child are devastating and are seen as a consequence of divorce and custody matters. Private and public law enforcement often view this matter as not something to concern themselves with. The report stresses that family abduction can be physically dangerous and sometimes as deadly for the child as any other form of child abduction (Office of Juvenile Justice and Delinquency Prevention, 2010).

Misperceptions about family abduction can promote further trauma to the child, increasing the frequency and duration of family abductions. Unfortunately, the worst part is the child's damage from the multifaceted diversity imperceptible to the naked eye, as it occurs deep within the child and lasts a lifetime (Office of Juvenile Justice and Delinquency Prevention, 2010). Divorce was mentioned in this study. However, SPA was not.

Child Abduction and Kidnapping in Australia

Of note is that some authors used the terms abduction and kidnapped interchangeably. For example, abduction and kidnapping are similar in that they involve taking someone against their will, but there is a subtle difference between them. Abduction is taking someone away by force or deception, often for a specific purpose, such as ransom, slavery, or sex trafficking. Abduction may also involve taking a child from one place to another without necessarily keeping them in confinement or using force during the abduction.

Kidnapping, on the other hand, involves taking a child by force, fraud, or deception with the intent to hold them captive, often for ransom or other demands. In addition, kidnapping typically involves holding the child in confinement or isolation and subjecting the victim to physical or emotional abuse. Subsequently, survivors may have experienced a further dimension: ' Child Abduction and Kidnapping' (Brown et al., 2014).

Under Australian law, abducting a child can also be viewed as kidnapping, which "is an offence under section 86 of the Crimes Act 1900 (NSW)" (Hickey & Nedim, 2020, p. 2). "Kidnapping carries a maximum penalty of 14 years in prison" (Hickey & Nedim, 2020, p. 2). To prove a kidnapping offence, the prosecution must demonstrate that: 1. A child was taken or detained, 2. the child was taken without the other person's consent, or 3. the intention was to hold the child to "ransom, or commit a serious indictable offence, or obtain any other advantage" (Hickey & Nedim, 2020, p. 2). A severe indictable offence is punishable by a minimum of five years in prison, including larceny (stealing). The maximum penalty may increase to twenty years if the kidnapper was in the company of another person/s or caused "actual bodily harm" to the child (Hickey & Nedim, 2020, p. 2). Actual bodily harm is also defined as more than "transient or trifling" and includes "lasting cuts and bruises" (Hickey & Nedim, 2020, p. 2).

Survivors may have been threatened with kidnapping (Baker, 2007, p. 88) and parental child abduction to make the alienated child think the parent was dangerous. For example, sometimes the APs tone became decidedly darker, and the children are led to believe that their TP is not safe and may inflict great harm on them through beatings, stories of plans of being aborted, thrown on a river, not caring for them properly or being kidnapped (Baker, 2007). Practitioners need to be aware that survivors may have experienced abduction or kidnapping by a family member, a friend of a family member, or an organisation specialising in the abduction or kidnapping of children involved in high-conflict divorce and SPA and will need to design therapy accordingly. Working with this population without extensive knowledge and expert clinical supervision is not recommended.

Post Divorce Kidnapping- A New Form of Child Abuse

Dorothy Huntington, a researcher and psychologist, observed a "simultaneous rise in the divorce rate and the incidence of post-divorce kidnapping" in 1986 and described this finding as "a new form of child abuse" (Lorandos et al., 2013, p.300). One example offered was the case of six-and-a-half-year-old twin girls who were abducted by their mother, aged forty, in 1995 after a "specific restraining order" was handed down by a Californian Court (Lorandos et al., 2013, p.404). During the divorce proceedings, the children were taken and held at the Mi'kmaq community reserve of Listuguj until March 1999. The children were indoctrinated to believe that judges were bad and that their father was a bad guy with a beard. After hearing all the evidence, the Court concluded that the children should be invested in the custody of their father, and they should rediscover the world outside of the community they had been kidnapped (Lorandos et al., 2013). Generalised divorce was mentioned in this study, but not PA or SPA.

Stockholm Syndrome, Kidnapping and PAS

The definition of Stockholm Syndrome is when someone who has been abducted or kidnapped is held for an extended period, and they begin to identify with their abductors/kidnappers (Berkowitz, n.d). The example given in Berkowitz (n.d) was when an heiress named Patti Hearst, whose family owned the Hearst Newspaper empire, was kidnapped and held hostage by the Symbionese Liberation Army (SLA) in 1974. After an extended period of living with her kidnappers, Patti began to identify with the plight of her captors and joined their cause. Patti did not want to be found or rescued. However, she was caught and returned home to years of intensive psychotherapy to deprogram her before she could return to everyday life (Berkowitz, n.d). The research reports that children of severe PAS show similarities to Patti Hearst and her programming (Baker, 1994).

Child Filicide, Suicide and Familicide

The inclusion of statistics on both step-parents and biological parents who commit filicide emphasises the urgency for further research and intervention to mitigate the detrimental effects of divorce and SPA on children and adult survivors. These statistics highlight the seriousness of the issue and underscore the need for comprehensive measures to prevent such tragic outcomes.

The world can be dangerous for children of SPA, SPAA, and SPA with kidnapping. The following section reports on another form of child maltreatment known as 'Child Filicide' (meaning the killing of children). The term 'Child Filicide' includes only the child or children being killed by one of their biological parents or step-parents (Brown et al., 2014). A second term known as 'Familicide' combined with 'Suicide' is where the child/children are killed, and the parent or step-parent dies by suicide after the act (Brown et al., 2014). 'Child Filicide' is an action that can occur in the context of high-conflict divorce and separation (Brown et al., 2014) and is a CIT that survivors may have been exposed to.

Forms of Parentification

Forms of parentification, known as emotional parentification and emotional incest, may also have occurred when the adult survivor was young. Parentification signifies a reversal of roles in a family where a child takes on adult parent responsibilities and is forced to meet the ongoing emotional needs required by their parent and siblings (Lo, 2019). The child also becomes the parent's counsellor, confidant, or emotional caretaker (Lo, 2019).

Emotional incest is a toxic dynamic known as covert incest (Lo, 2019). It involves the parent looking toward the child for the connection and support they usually receive from a partner (Lo, 2019). They may also become an intimate partner to the parent where the parent may display sexualised behaviours, abuse the child, or become emotionally suffocating (Lo, 2019). The parent may also cry excessively in front of the child, talk about being sexually frustrated, sleep with the child or adolescent in the same bed (sometimes to avoid intimacy with their partner) and make sexual remarks about the adolescent's developing body (Lo, 2019).

Consequently, the child or adolescent may also feel guilty if they want to be left alone, experience feelings of enmeshment, and often feel obligated to meet the needs and whims expressed by the parent (Lo, 2019). Many survivors in Baker's (2007) study reported experiencing sexual or physical abuse by the AP or their step-parents. In addition, survivors stated that their AP often used emotionally manipulative strategies such as creating loyalty binds, cultivating dependency, and withdrawing love (Baker, 2007).

PA is considered a form of emotional abuse for the following reasons. Early research explains that the strategies used by the AP to effectuate the alienation process are emotionally abusive due to the verbal assaults experienced by the child and the corruption levels (Baker, 2007). Also described were the terror experienced, being overly pressured to conform, the experience of rejection if there is nonconformity and the isolation of the child from the TP (Baker, 2007). The survivors in these studies also described emotionally abusive brainwashing techniques they were exposed to in the form of thinking in black and white and negative statements regarding their TP (Baker, 2007). This early research suggested separating a child from their parent signifies emotional abuse. This study also mentioned PA as having long-reaching effects and co-occurring with other forms of maltreatment, such as alcoholism and personality disorders in the AP.

The Long-Term Effects of SPA

Abandonment and Attachment

Previous research states that the experience of SPA stays with the child into adulthood, and practitioners often do not recognise the complex trauma of attachment and abandonment (Childress, 2015). Therefore, the key concepts of attachment and abandonment for survivors are described in the following sections.

Strategies of attachment and alienation were reported in early studies where researchers interpreted the stories mentioned by the survivors through the lens of attachment theory (Bowlby, 1980). Tactics described by the survivors that came from their APs were reported as practical strategies that interfered with the "developing or existing attachment relationship between the adult child of PAS (as a child) and the targeted parent" (Baker, 2007, p. 107).

Bowlby (1980) posits that losing a loved one is among the most excruciatingly painful experiences a person can endure. To the bereaved, true comfort can only come from the return of the lost individual. Anything less is often perceived as an insult (Bowlby, 1980). In his 1960 paper, "Grief and Mourning in Infancy and Early Childhood," Bowlby (1980, p. 15) drew attention to the remarkable resemblances between young children's reactions to losing their mother and those of grieving adults. Additionally, Bowlby observed that the mourning responses observed in infancy and early childhood often exhibit several features typical of pathological mourning in adults. (Bowlby, 1980).

Dr Elisabeth Kubler-Ross (1969) created historical, pioneering research proposing that there were "five stages in coming to terms with death: denial, anger, bargaining, depression and acceptance" (Mahmood, 2006, p. 232). These five stages were developed after Dr Kubler-Ross (1969) spoke with 500 terminally ill patients. According to earlier grief research, grief and mourning are closely linked to individuals who have experienced the death of a loved one. In many cultures, conventional forms of mourning behaviour are practised to unite people and help them transition through the grieving process as a community (Mahmood, 2006). In the case of one study participant and survivor of SPAA, "Aurora", who had been abducted from her beloved TP at an early age, shared;

> Sometimes, it felt as though my alienated father had died, and I didn't know if he had died when I was young. After forty-four years, I finally reunited with him, and he died two years later. I had the same lot of grief come flooding back, but I could go through the grief stages the second time. It's a constant state of grief that never ends. It feels like he has died twice." (Aurora)

Loss and Attachment

Early research explains that the PAS survivors' inability to experience the grieving stages when TP leaves are associated with depression and consequent relational problems (Baker, 2007). Loss is also a prevalent feature for survivors of PA and can come in the form of a "cascade of losses" that can include the "loss of individual self," "loss of childhood and innocence," "loss of a good enough parent," "loss of extended family," "loss of community," and the "interconnectedness of loss" (Harman et al., 2021, pp. 6-9).

In a study focused on the British-Indian survivors of divorce by Das (2016), survivors described the emotional consequences of their parent's divorce as having experienced feelings of sadness and loss, loss of a parent, loss of experiences, loss of childhood, loss of freedom and loss of possibilities. Bowlby's early research into loss and attachment explained how children between twelve months and three years of age respond when separated from the mother figure to whom they are attached and placed with strangers in a strange place (Bowlby, 1980). Bowlby noted that through his work, the text often referred to the caregiver by the term 'mother', but he wanted the reader to understand that he also referred to a person who mothers a child and becomes attached.

Another example described in Bowlby's historic research explained that one child's initial response was to protest loudly and make an "urgent effort" to rejoin his mother (Bowlby, 1980, p. 9). This behaviour includes periods where the child was emotionally up and down for a week or more, combined with periods of feeling "buoyed up" with the expectation and hopes that his mother would return soon and he would not be abandoned (Bowlby, 1980, p. 9). Not long after, despair set in. Despite the hope fading, he became apathetic and withdrawn, and his mother's longing did not diminish. Consequently, a realisation stage had begun (Bowlby, 1980). His despair was only broken by an "intermittent and monotonous wail" during a "state of unutterable misery" (Bowlby, 1980, p. 9).

Abandonment is a common theme among survivors, and 'threatening abandonment' was an experience mentioned by survivors that their alienators had used to abuse them in earlier research (Baker, 2007). For a child threatened with abandonment, a deep-seated fear that they are unworthy, unsafe and may be uncared for is deeply instilled (Baker, 2007). Loss and abandonment were common themes during the childhoods of the survivors in Baker's (2007) study, especially if they expressed a desire to contact their TP.

Some examples of abandonment threats described by the survivors who requested to see their TP were, "You can go live on the street with your father," "I'll kick you out," "You are not going to see him, and if you mention his name you're out." Also described were, "You kids are pieces of crap. You're just like him, and it is time for you to go. I am going to try to find him, and you are gone" (Baker, 2007, p. 156).

Abandonment is a common theme among survivors. However, other forms of divorce and SPA-related CITs present more serious challenges.

These include the shooting, kidnap and torture of a child, child filicide, and suicide and familicide, where the perpetrator kills the entire family before taking their own life (Brown et al., 2014), as explained in the following topics:

The Long-Term Effects of SPA and Traumatic Violent Events

Shooting, Kidnap and Torture

The community faces even more significant difficulties when dealing with divorce and SPA linked to traumatic events such as shooting, kidnapping, and torturing a child (University of the Health Sciences, 2021). Three toxic factors differentiating the traumatic events of the shooting, kidnapping, and torturing of a child from other forms of SPA violence are: 1. The child is usually held against their will. 2. The injury to the child had been intentionally thought about and personally directed. 3. Pain on the child is inflicted for punishment, penetration, pleasure, or coercion (University of the Health Sciences, 2021).

Furthermore, survivors of coercive trauma may develop psychiatric disorders after their exposure to trauma. Therefore, it is recommended that psychiatric screening of all children who have been through this level of trauma have periodical check-ups for emotional reactions that will ensure that symptoms are identified early to assist in a long-term promotion of health outcomes for when they turn into survivors of trauma (University of the Health Sciences, 2021).

Understanding Filicide, Suicide, and Familicide Amid Separation, Divorce, and Custody Disputes

Child homicide is described as the intentional killing of a child or infant and is a rare yet alarming occurrence that commands community and media attention (Johnson, 2008). The terms filicide, infanticide, and neonaticide have been used interchangeably in child homicide studies (Debowska et al., 2015, p. 114). In Australia, several high-profile cases involved the murder of a child or children by their biological parent or male step-parent, many of which happened within the framework of divorce and separation. For example, in some cases, motives for filicide, or filicide, familicide and suicide followed a legal dispute about parenting, succeeding the divorce. However, little information is available about the perpetrators' background or why they committed the offence (Johnson, 2008).

Historical research by Resnick (1969) and Scott (1973) explains that a child murderer's origin of aggression derives from a displaced partner, parent or sibling and then directed at a more vulnerable target such as a child (Resnick, 1969; Scott, 1973). Furthermore, according to previous research, displaced aggression theory suggests that if a person cannot express their aggression directly toward the source of provocation, they may transfer it onto an innocent individual or object (Anderson & Bushman, 2002). Therefore, practitioners interested in comprehending the processes that contribute to filicide are advised to consider the framework of family dynamics. (Debowska et al., 2015).

Early studies reported that filicide might have been gendered, but this has been refuted by later studies that refer to "gender being a factor in different kinds of filicide deaths" (Bourget et al., 2007; Grace & Whitehurst, 2007; Kirkwood, 2012; Putkonen et al., 2011). A ten-year study on the findings of filicide in Victoria, Australia, from selected files within the Victorian Coroner's Office between 2000-2009 examined whether separation, divorce, domestic violence, and mental illness were elements in these cases (Brown et al., 2014). These studies aimed to fill the gap within existing Australian research. However, the researchers discovered that the findings were similar to research in the United Kingdom that reported that the understandings of perpetrators who had killed a child were highly complex, especially in conjunction with developing a psychological or relationship problem in their lifetime (Stroud, 2008). The study examined whether filicide perpetrators had been in contact with family and friends, support services, MHPs, general practitioners and child protection services. The key messages from the study reported that while there is a mounting body of evidence examining filicide in cases of parental separation and divorce (Johnson, 2005; Mouzos & Rushforth, 2003), Australia lacks a comprehensive examination of filicide cases (Alder & Polk, 2001; Strang, 1996). In support of international evidence, research conducted in Canada supported the evidence that parental separation is linked to filicide deaths (Bourget et al., 2007).

A study by Lewis and Bunce (2003) reported significant differences between mothers who commit filicide with or without mental illness concerning maternal history, demographic variables, behavioural patterns, and offence characteristics before and after the murder of their child. The study found that the group of psychotic women (*n*=29), who compared to non-psychotic women (*n*=26), were older, more likely to have been married, separated, or divorced, achieved higher levels of education, were less likely to be employed and often had a history of substance abuse and suicide attempts. Women in the filicide group were also more likely to have previously been sexually abused and physically abused (Lewis & Bunce, 2003). Domestic violence was measured between the two groups of women, and no group differences were noted (Debowska et al., 2015). With regard to this study, four MHP study participants reported working with the complex issue of familicide and homicide among adult survivors of SPA. Please refer to Familicide and Homicide SPA Complex Intersecting Traumas Reported to MHPs in Volume Two.

Traumagenic Model of Childhood Sexual Abuse

Finkelhor and Brown's (1985) 'traumagenic model' theoretical framework explains how clients who experience CSA may live with consequences later in life. The model proposes four trauma-causing dynamics within the experience of understanding CSA: traumatic sexualisation, powerlessness, betrayal, and the effect of stigmatisation. Adult survivors who experience these dynamics have their emotional and cognitive picture of the world altered by distortion of their affective capacities, self-concept, and worldview. For example, the dynamic stigmatisation changes a child's sense of their value. For MHPs who work with survivors, the symptoms of SPA, combined with CSA, must also be considered.

Traumatic Sexualisation

The traumatic sexualisation dynamic describes a "process in which a child's sexuality (including both sexual feelings and sexual attitudes) is shaped in a developmentally inappropriate and interpersonally dysfunctional fashion as a result of sexual abuse" (Finkelhor & Browne, 1985, p. 531)

Powerlessness

The powerlessness dynamic interferes with a child's sensibility to control their lives. Children who try and cope with the world from within these dynamics may display behavioural problems that have been commonly noticed in CSA victims (Finkelhor & Browne, 1985).

Betrayal

Finkelhor and Browne (1985, p. 531) define betrayal as "the dynamic by which children discover that someone on whom they were vitally dependent has caused them harm".

Dissociation and Abuse

The term 'dissociation' describes a range of experiences that an adult survivor of abuse may display, ranging from mild detachment from their immediate environment to severe detachment, which is not the same as a total loss of reality from physical or emotional experience (Briere J. N., 1992). In addition, research on the long-term sequelae of childhood sexual abuse reports that various psychosocial problems are more common among adult survivors than others with no such abuse (Briere

& Runtz, 1993). Various CSA-related problems are listed under the categories of cognitive distortions, stress disorder, altered emotionality (depression and anxiety), avoidance (substance abuse, suicidality, and tension-reducing activities), dissociative phenomena (manifestation of depersonalisation, disengagement, out-of-body experiences, (Briere & Runtz, 1987), (Putnam, 1985, as cited in Briere & Runtz, 1993) disturbed relatedness and impaired self-reference (Briere & Runtz, 1993).

Domestic Violence and Filicide

The connection between filicide, the tragic act of killing one's own child, and domestic violence has been identified through extensive research carried out by FDV and death review committees (Jaffe et al., 2013; Martin & Pritchard, 2010) and from the findings associated to the deaths of children who were under the care of state child protection services (Jaffe et al., 2012). Findings for domestic violence linked to filicide were reported as understated because after a child has been killed, the focus is on the data collected about the child's death, not the domestic violence they were involved in. This fact, combined with the circumstance that domestic violence is often secret and is often not reported in families, may have skewed the data (Brown et al., 2014).

Divorce and Separation as Contributing Factors of Filicide

Previous Australian research by Johnson (2008) reports that the experience of separation and divorce can be exceptionally challenging and protracted, lasting for numerous years. Furthermore, Johnson (2008) emphasises that individuals' actions in such circumstances are primarily influenced by their subjective perceptions of their relationship rather than solely relying on objective facts.

Furthermore, building upon Johnson's perspective, a study conducted by Brown et al. (2014) reported that half of the participants (n=23) in their study had been exposed to parental divorce and separation. The study findings highlighted a challenging reality, as the number encompassed 12 cases where the mother killed the children, nine children their father killed, and two children and two instances where the stepfather committed the crime (Brown et al., 2014). In addition, for 17 of the victims, the parents had recently been separated, stating that this was a contributing factor, and for the remaining five, their parent's separation had not been recent (Brown et al., 2014).

Statistics on Stepparents and Biological Parents Who Commit Filicide

The study also reported that "stepfathers killed children mostly in the one-to-four-year age group," and there was minimal difference between the sexes of the children killed (Brown et al., 2014, p. 83). "Biological mothers killed male children at three times the rate of female children" and were most likely to kill children under one. (Brown et al., 2014, p. 83). Biological mothers also killed considerable numbers of children in the one to four age group (N=6). However, they were less likely to kill older children and "did not kill any children over the age of 14 years" (Brown et al., 2014, p. 83). Biological fathers were reported as killing children under one more frequently and children aged one to four less frequently. Biological fathers killed male children at "three times the rate of female children (11 compared to 4)" (Brown et al., 2014, p. 83). Finally, children aged between 15 and 18 were only killed by their biological fathers (Brown et al., 2014).

Suicide and Familicide Associated with Filicide

The previously described study also reported that single filicide deaths were listed as the most common out of the participants (n=24 children), with a notable gap between single and multiple deaths by filicide (n=5 children). Single filicide and suicide deaths were reported (n=4 children), and this number occurred as often as multiple filicide and suicide (n=4 children), and lastly, familicide (n=3 children) was reported at (n=3 children). Thus, a little over half the deaths of children in the study were attributed to a single filicide perpetrated by a biological parent who did not die by suicide at the time (Brown et al., 2014).

Mental Illness

Filicide

The study reported a variety of mental illnesses that were identified among the perpetrators. Depression was found among 59.3% of all perpetrators and paranoid schizophrenia was ranked second (18.5%). Following on were obsessive-compulsive disorder (3.7%) and a variety of other diagnoses such as psychosis (11.1%), nervous breakdown (7.4%), suicidal ideation (11.1%), irrational violence behaviour (3.7%), homicidal ideation (3.7%) and mood swings (3.7%) (Brown et al., 2014). This research indicated that medical professionals did not follow up on the assessments for homicidal and suicidal ideation made after checking the child's safety in filicide cases (Brown et al., 2014).

Mental Illness, Divorce and Separation as Factors of Filicide

The study suggests several stress factors that may increase the chances of filicide in families. Mental illness (particularly depression) combined with parental divorce and separation was the most commonly linked factor for fathers and mothers to kill their children. For stepfathers, parental divorce and separation were not linked in the same way but rather an underlying factor that promoted their entry into the family. Mental illness was reported as an associated factor for biological fathers and mothers but not so much for stepfathers (Brown et al., 2014).

Finally, the psychosocial approach and related parallel traumas utilised in this chapter shed light on the prevalence of filicide in Australia, where an average of 5.7 children were killed annually by their biological fathers, mothers, and stepfathers. The chapter identified mental illness, particularly depression, divorce, and separation, as common factors across all groups. Although family violence and substance abuse were less prevalent, stepfathers were frequently associated with these factors. However, these studies did not examine filicide concerning stepmothers or other forms, such as stranger-perpetrated filicide. The chapter underscores the need for further research to understand better the international parallels and intervention strategies to combat filicide. These studies did not address the impact of SPA on children or adults who may have been exposed to filicide, suicide, and familicide.

Researchers' Note to MHPs Regarding Survivors of SPA and Filicide

This chapter examined the relationship between SPA and various psychological factors, including dissociation, identity disorders, and other outcomes. The study sought to understand how PA contributes to developing these psychological consequences. These studies highlight the importance for MHPs, mental health professionals and medical professionals to consider whether survivors may have been exposed to the related CITs discussed in this chapter.

All professionals, especially MHPs, are encouraged to remain vigilant and aware of the potential for survivors of SPA to have been threatened with or overheard conversations about filicide or suicide being planned for them or have come close to experiencing such incidents themselves but were intercepted. It is also possible that survivors may have experienced such incidents directly but survived the attack and may still carry the memories from these events. For example, they may see themselves as having lived through a near-death experience (such as "Aurora" in these studies) and be reliving the event and potentially recovering from the physical injuries inflicted upon them. Alternatively, it may have happened to a sibling or other family member, such as their biological mother or father. Therefore, it is crucial for MHPs to assess the potential impact of these traumatic experiences on child or adult survivors and to provide appropriate support and interventions to address any resulting psychological distress.

Conclusion

In conclusion, the various topics covered in this list highlight the devastating impact of SPA and divorce on child and adult survivors. SPA and related forms of emotional abuse are explored as contributing factors to trauma and abuse within families, particularly in the context of divorce and separation. Child abduction, filicide, suicide, and familicide are also discussed as potential outcomes of SPA and the long-term effects of emotional and physical abuse.

Furthermore, the statistics on step-parents and biological parents who commit filicide demonstrate the need for further research and intervention strategies to address the impact of divorce and SPA on survivors and their families. By describing these critical aspects, the Researcher has established a link between SPA and violence-related psychological outcomes. The data emphasises the necessity for continued research, intervention, and support to address the profound impact of divorce and SPA on survivors and their communities.

Chapter Three

An Extended Literature Review

The recognition and appropriate treatment of trauma experienced by survivors is an ethical responsibility for MHPs. However, existing findings suggest that many MHPs lack the necessary training and tools to address the needs of this population effectively. This lack of recognition raises significant questions regarding the professional responsibility of the mental health field to bridge this training and practice gap. Consequently, there is a critical gap in the professional training of practitioners in this field, resulting in survivors experiencing unaddressed social, physical, and mental health challenges. This gap not only hinders the provision of adequate support and intervention for survivors of SPA, but it also poses ethical concerns regarding the well-being of these individuals.

These studies adopted an exploratory approach by examining the peer-reviewed and grey literature and identifying the perceived knowledge gaps. The Researcher extended the literature review to bridge research knowledge gaps and effectively address the needs of SPA survivors. The main and sub-questions of the research are offered again as a reminder for the reader as follows:

Main Question

1. What are the perspectives of adult survivors of SPA and the MHPs who work with them to address the symptoms of SPA during therapy?

Sub Questions

1a. What are the perspectives of adult survivors of SPA regarding their consultations with MHPs during and or after therapy to treat symptoms pertaining to SPA?

1b. What are the perspectives of MHPs who work with adult survivors of SPA pertaining to their symptomology?

This chapter does not solely focus on addressing the research questions outlined due to a lack of current information and research specifically dedicated to the professional training and practices of MHPs in working with survivors of SPA. As a result, the literature review cast a wide net and branched out into various related parallel trauma areas to gather insights and fill the knowledge gap. The additional areas explored in this chapter include examining peer-reviewed articles on family therapy programs, recommended websites and blogs, a study on adverse outcomes of divorce, and an Australian study on adult children of PA. Significantly few articles were discovered in this comprehensive search.

As a result of the initial academic peer-reviewed search yielding limited information, a thorough investigation was conducted on the grey literature pertaining to divorce, PA, and SPA. The exploration of grey literature also investigated resources for emergency help related to SPA and the lack of professional knowledge on SPA. The review also provides a summary of current treatment approaches for MHPs to address PA and SPA, including individual and family therapy interventions. Considering these extended areas, the extended review offers a comprehensive exploration of the topic, enabling a better understanding of the dynamics and CITs associated with SPA in a field where there has not been much research thus far. The grey literature review is reported after the peer-reviewed content.

Peer-Reviewed Literature

A peer-reviewed extended literature search was conducted using reputable databases such as MEDLINE, APA PsycNet, and Psychiatry Online. The following contents present the design and search strategy, followed by divorce studies, family therapy programs and relevant studies on adverse outcomes. Furthermore, Australian research on adult children of PA and a study on Italian college students' exposure to PA is reported.

Keywords

The Researcher developed eleven search terms deemed suitable to discover relevant published literature covering "adult survivors of severe parental alienation" and "mental health practitioners". These search terms were: "Parental Alienation", "Parental Alienation" AND "ACEs", "Parental Alienation" AND "Adult", "Parental Alienation" AND "Adult Children", "Parental Alienation" AND "Anxiety", "Parental Alienation" AND "Child Abuse", "Parental Alienation" AND "Conflict", "Parental Alienation" AND "Depression", "Parental Alienation" AND "Mental Health Practitioners", "Parental Alienation" AND "Parental Conflict", "Parental Alienation" AND "Therapists". The Researcher used these eleven search terms to query three electronic academic databases. These databases were MEDLINE, APA PsycNet, and Psychiatry Online.

These keywords were selected because they reflected the study's focus on the impact of SPA on adult survivors, the mental health consequences, and the involvement of MHPs in treating survivors. Additionally, the inclusion of the keywords "adverse childhood experiences" aimed to capture relevant literature that explored the broader context of childhood trauma and its potential influence on the psychological well-being of survivors of SPA.

Furthermore, throughout the extended literature review, the Researcher modified the initial keywords slightly if no results were located. For example, if the term 'mental health practitioner' returned no results, the term 'mental health professional' would be substituted. None of the slightly changed keywords reported any results either. This detailed change was performed to ensure a more targeted search and identify distinct sets of keywords that yielded relevant results. The results obtained from the clusters of keywords were utilised for subsequent investigations, allowing for a comprehensive exploration of the literature on MHPs treating survivors of PA.

Peer-Reviewed Article Search Strategy

The Researcher extensively reviewed the existing literature to locate pertinent peer-reviewed articles. The main aim of the extensive literature review was to explore the body of published works focusing on adult survivors of SPA and the therapeutic treatment approaches employed by MHPs working with this population.

The inclusion criteria for studies to be included in the literature review were as follows:

1. Peer-reviewed journal articles published in English between 2016 and 2021.
2. Articles that provided information about studies related to working with adult survivors of SPA regarding treatment protocols used by MHPs.

To ensure the accuracy and rigour of the screening process, a blind review was conducted by an independent PhD researcher who was not involved in the initial search and screening process. This additional researcher was responsible for overseeing the review and verifying the inclusion and exclusion decisions made by the primary researcher. During the blind review, the independent researcher was provided with the list of articles that passed the initial screening based on titles and abstracts. The independent reviewer was briefed on the primary researcher's specific inclusion and exclusion criteria. The independent researcher carefully assessed each article based on its title and abstract, comparing it against the inclusion and exclusion criteria established for the study. This blind review aimed to minimise bias and ensure that the final selection of articles for the peer-reviewed literature review was as objective and accurate as possible. Any discrepancies or disagreements between the primary Researcher and the independent reviewer regarding the inclusion or exclusion of specific articles were resolved through discussion and consensus. This collaborative approach helped maintain the integrity and reliability of the literature review process.

Peer-Reviewed Literature Database Results

The Researcher performed 33 searches, with only four of the searches yielding nil results, resulting in a combined 3,923 results from the remaining 29 searches. The total results were then filtered to remove any article that appeared in the list more than once. This produced 788 unique articles. The list of unique articles was further refined by applying a filter that excluded all articles published before 2016, resulting in a final set of 88 articles. All searches were recorded on an Excel spreadsheet. All of the articles were individually reviewed and eliminated if the title or abstract did not meet the inclusion criteria. All 88 articles of the final set were excluded because these articles focused exclusively on children and did not mention either 'adult survivors of severe parental alienation' or the treatment protocols used by MHPs.

It is worth noting that despite efforts to remove duplicates within each database, some duplicates across the chosen databases could not be eliminated completely. For example, special characters within abstracts, possibly introduced during formatting or copying, led to some duplicates within the PsychNet database. To address this, abstracts were hand-edited to remove the special characters.

The final step involved further screening the remaining articles based on their titles and abstracts to determine their relevance for inclusion in the study. This screening process was guided by the specific inclusion and exclusion criteria, ensuring that only articles meeting the research objectives were considered. No articles were found in any of the peer-reviewed academic databases.

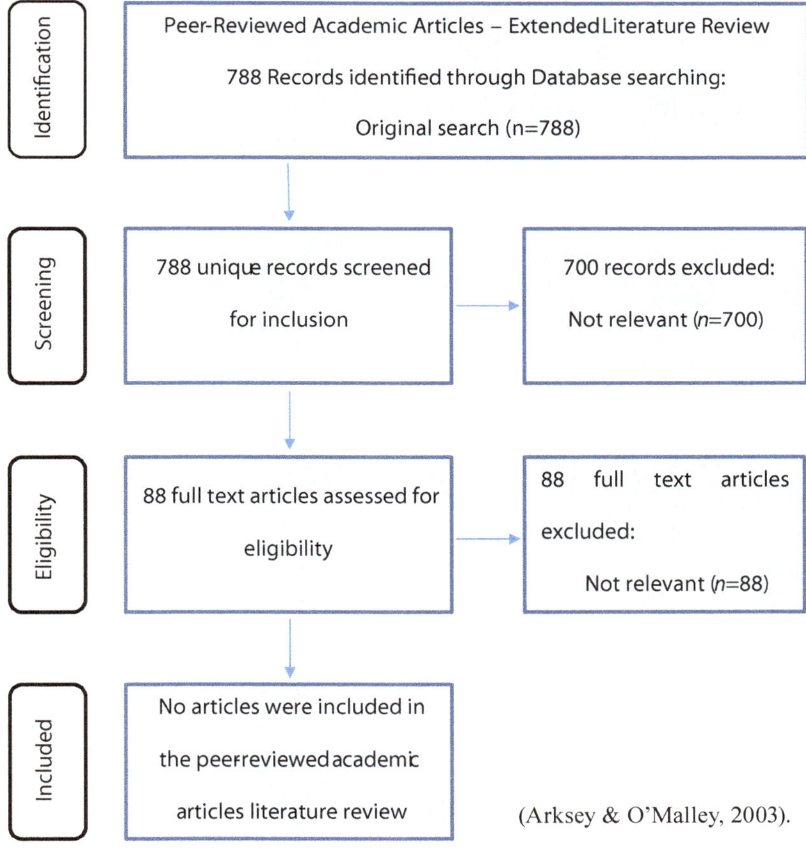

(Arksey & O'Malley, 2003).

FIGURE ONE

Results-PRISMA Flowchart of Peer-Reviewed Academic Articles

Peer-Reviewed Articles Reporting on Family Therapy Programmes

These studies discovered that current peer-reviewed articles reporting on treatments available to MHPs working with survivors are sparse. Therefore, a systematic review by Templer et al. (2016) reporting on children of PA, not SPA, is discussed as a related parallel study. This study was chosen as it summarises the literature regarding best practices for practitioners who work with children of PA. However, this study was not included in the Prisma results diagram as it did not fall into these studies' criteria for inclusion.

The systematic review of the literature regarding PA to determine best practices for therapists and legal practitioners identified a selection of specialised family therapy programmes for children. Previous research has indicated that these programs share a common objective while utilising various delivery methods (Templer et al., 2016). Specifically, family therapy programs involve the participation of the targeted child, TP, and AP, who receive psychoeducation and therapeutic interventions from practitioners.

In addition, conflict resolution, establishing healthy boundaries and techniques that challenge the distorted thinking of the child and AP are also included (Templer et al., 2016). However, there is no mention of where the MHPs have received their training or how these practitioners apply these protocols to children of PA. Costings were not included for the family therapy programmes described. However, individual therapy costs were mentioned and ranged from $150 to $325 (USD) per hour.

The systematic review has uncovered a pressing need for rigorous, empirically tested treatment protocols to be developed for practitioners who work with survivors. These protocols are necessary because the SPA phenomenon is highly complex and largely misunderstood by practitioners. For example, Morgan and colleagues (2020) highlight the lack of evidence in academic reports, commentary papers and publications regarding interventions for PA (Morgan et al., 2020). Further, the previous research focus has tended to be on children and has not extended very far into how the child's well-being or mental health is affected in adulthood.

Grey Literature Extended Literature Review

Search Strategy

Due to the limited information available on SPA within the peer-reviewed literature and the academic databases, the Researcher undertook a comprehensive extended literature review of the grey literature. Following the Arksey and O'Malley (2003) framework, the Researcher decided to encompass children and adults involved in intervention or treatment programs targeting mild to severe PA. The extended literature review aimed to capture and review current interventions and treatment protocols utilised with this population.

On January 11th, 2022, an extended literature review of grey literature was conducted using a framework influenced by (Pham et al., 2014). The databases were selected based on their comprehensiveness and coverage of various disciplines related to PA. The Researcher adopted a thematic review approach, meticulously collecting information from various sources for the grey literature searches. These sources encompassed books on PA and SPA available in Australia, grey literature databases, Google listings, websites, and PA blogs. Any potential literature was analysed according to the title and first two paragraphs to determine eligibility for inclusion. The findings were diligently recorded by hand and systematically added to the corresponding sections under each theme or category.

This comprehensive thematic review explored multiple aspects of SPA treatment protocols, including current interventions and treatment protocols for children and adult survivors. Additionally, the Researcher investigated the availability of reunification hotels/camps, SPA course curriculums, associated costs of therapy or treatment programs, therapists' qualifications, training, case consultation, and related resources for practitioners. By integrating the findings into the thematic framework, the Researcher ensured a structured and cohesive analysis, enhancing the overall clarity and coherence of the grey literature review.

Grey Literature Criteria

Inclusion Criteria

1. Grey literature articles from books available in Australia, databases, websites, and blogs printed in English relating to psychological interventions for mild to severe parental alienation (no dates applied).
2. Grey literature articles or information about program interventions and treatment protocols for children and adult survivors of mild to severe PA.

Exclusion Criteria

1. Articles that are academic and/or peer-reviewed.
2. Articles that did not mention parental alienation, parental conflict, SPA, child, adult, treatment, therapy, intervention, custody, or divorce.
3. Articles describing hypothetical examples or directly related to divorce with no reference to children or adults who have experienced mild to severe PA.
4. Articles that mention treatment for children experiencing PA and CSA sent to Deprogramming Camps, Boarding Schools, Boot Camps, Wilderness Camps, or Residential Treatment Centres.

Results from the grey literature review are presented in Figure Two, titled 'Results. PRISMA Flowchart of Grey Literature Extended Literature Review' in this chapter.

The thorough exploration of grey literature databases and sources employed four different searches: (1) exploration of grey literature books focusing on parental alienation and severe parental alienation available for purchase, (2) searches within grey literature databases, including The Australian Institute of Family Studies, The Australian Institute of Health and Welfare, Emerald Insight, and employing the 'All Newspapers' option, (3) customised Google searches, and (4) targeted examination of relevant websites and blogs.

The grey literature searches were sourced from books on PA and SPA available in Australia, grey literature databases, Google listings, websites, and PA blogs and added to Excel spreadsheets. In addition, the grey literature extended literature review examined which current interventions, treatment protocols, and reunification hotels/camps are available for children and survivors. Also searched were SPA course curriculums, the cost associated with the therapy or treatment program for survivors, the qualifications of the person/people administering the therapy, and what training, case consultation, and related costs practitioners can access.

The Researcher designed the extended literature review to follow a structured approach to identify existing interventions and treatment protocols for child and adult survivors of mild to severe PA, consisting of three key steps: (1) Conducting a comprehensive systematic search of the grey literature, including books, databases, websites, and blogs, (2) Analysing and summarising the characteristics and variety of interventions and treatment protocols identified, and (3) Examining the reported challenges and limitations associated with these interventions and treatment protocols, following the framework outlined by Pham et al. (2014).

Given that search engines and databases use unique algorithms to produce their relevant rating schemes, the Researcher decided that combining these sources would likely lead to a broader range of articles (Godin et al., 2015).

Grey Literature Search Results

The combined first search of the grey literature found on Google, namely PA websites and PA website blogs, identified 19,788,022 records. Two 'Recommended to Researcher' websites and 24 books that mentioned 'children, adults, PA and SPA' were screened for inclusion. A total of 19,787,999 results emerged from the first and second combined searches. Furthermore, 19,787,999 records were screened and excluded due to not meeting the study criteria. Not relevant (*n*=19,787,999). A reduced total of 49 mentions were identified and screened for inclusion. This figure of 49 was screened again and consequently reduced to twenty-three full electronic articles assessed for final eligibility, plus two books and one 'Recommended to Researcher' website.

Grey Literature Books

The grey literature book search produced two results out of twenty-four written for MHPs. The first result was Childress's book, 'An Attachment-Based Model of Parental Alienation (ABPA)- Foundations (2015). This book offers MHP's training in PA and SPA. However, Dr Childress refers to this phenomenon as 'attachment-based parental alienation.' Dr Childress is a licensed clinical psychologist in California, America. In his book, Dr Childress explains what is involved regarding ABPA at the family systems level, the personality disorder level, and the attachment system level (Childress, 2015, p. 1). Issues faced by mental health professionals include diagnosis, treatment, and professional competence required when working with SPA clients (Childress, 2015, p. 1). The cost of training for MHPs is not mentioned in this book. Dr Childress' qualifications as a clinical psychologist were verified.

The second resource was a website also by Childress (2020) that provides mental health professionals with free and comprehensive resources for working with child and adult survivors of mild to severe ABPA (Childress, 2015). Additionally, Childress offered a clinical supervision program for MHPs, available at a service fee and conducted on a six-monthly basis. Dr Childress reports having extensive experience working with survivors of PA and SPA, targeted and APs. His clinical services are $250 (USD) per hour.

The second book result was Restoring Family Connections by (Baker et al., 2020). This book offers a how-to guide for licensed mental health professionals who work with TPs and their adult children of PA. The authors' qualifications state that Baker is a developmental psychologist, Fine is a licensed clinical social worker, and Lacheen-Baker is a licensed practical nurse. The Researcher verified Bakers' and Fines' qualifications; however, Lacheen-Bakers' qualifications could not be verified.

Baker et al. (2020) explain that treatments are available elsewhere for families affected by PA but are not readily available. This program offers "theoretical principles of PA", "Restoring Family Connections Preprogram Sessions", and 'In and Out of Session Activities" (Baker et al., 2020, p. 5). Testimonials were sourced from professionals with an understanding of PA. No testimonials were recorded from older children or TPs who had been through the programme. Costs were not recommended.

Database Search

The Researcher searched four grey literature databases to find information on interventions and protocols for child and adult survivors of PA and SPA. However, no relevant results were found using the keywords "parental alienation," "child," "treatment program," and "reunification program."

Google Search

During the grey literature search using the Google keyword "reunification camp*," six results were found regarding interventions for children who have experienced PA and SPA. This section focused on the most relevant findings. For instance, one of the searches led to Turning Points for Families, located in Texas, USA. The organisers offer an intensive four-day treatment program for families dealing with SPA. The program is overseen by Loretta Maase (MA, LPC-S) and her associates (Turning Points for Families, 2014).

A second article about Friedlander and Walters' 'Multimodal Family Intervention' advertises reunification therapy with varying interventions for parental alignment, enmeshment, alienation, and estrangement (Huesch, 2019). In addition, the Family Bridges Program for Alienated Children (FBAC), recently renamed The Family Bridges Workshop FBW (Korosi, 2022), is promoted as a court-mandated reunification therapy camp and was also included in the article on Friedlander and Walters by Huesch (2019). The FBAC programme is advertised as evidence-based and run by accredited facilitators providing family consultants, single expert witnesses and legal counsel before the Family Court (Korosi, 2017). The FBAC in Australia is administered by Korosi (PhD), a certified psychotherapist and administrative services director. Dr Korosi's qualifications have been verified.

The third article, written by Kruk (PhD), was discovered on the Child Rights Foundation website. In this article, Kruk (2022) emphasises the importance of involving service providers with specialised expertise in reuniting parentally alienated children when undertaking reunification efforts after a prolonged absence. Kruk also mentions the FBAC program and highlights Sullivan's Overcoming Barriers Family Camp (Sullivan et al., 2010). The Overcoming Barriers article advertises a program that combines psycho-educational and clinical intervention within a milieu therapy environment, aimed at facilitating the development of a parenting time agreement and a written aftercare plan (Kruk, 2022).

The fourth listing reported that Jones (a child and family therapist) and Associates (2022) run the' The Family Forward Reunification Therapy and Counselling Program'. This website advertises that they offer a unique program that is given referrals by the Court system to establish "appropriate, healthy child-parent relationships" (Family Forward Reunification Therapy and Counselling Program, 2022, p. 1).

The fifth listing consisted of an article by the family lawyer Isicoff (2019), focusing on PA and reunification therapy. Isicoff (2019) promotes an 'outpatient approach therapy' specifically designed for moderate to severely alienated children. The program, known as "The Stable Paths Approach," utilises a treatment model developed by Transitioning Families, a California-based program that claims to have successfully conducted reunification workshops since 2006 (Isicoff, 2019, p. 1). The activities offered in this program include horse exercises, recreational sports, swimming with dolphins, cooking meals together, playing games, rebuilding existing bonds, and creating new memories (Isicoff, 2019). Unfortunately, the Stable Paths website (Doelz, 2021) did not provide further information regarding PA, reunification programs, staff qualifications or associated costs.

Lastly, one other website named "Time to Put Kids First" included the keywords "reunification camp" (Time to Put Kids First, 2019). This website states that they offer various services and programs to educate the public and equip parents with tools for success. While no specific costs were listed for the reunification camp, the website provided several donation options. Additionally, there were sections where visitors could subscribe to their newsletter.

Websites and Blogs Recommended to the Researcher

As part of the Researcher's investigation, colleagues recommended searching websites and blogs. One of the recommended sources was The Conscious Co-Parenting Institute, which promotes the 'High Road to Reunification Program' facilitated by Pruter (ND), who serves as the CEO/Founder of CCPI. This program aims to break the cycle of abuse and rebuild a loving bond between parent and child through a transformative workshop that creates a safe environment for both (Conscious Co-Parenting Institute, 2022). In the blog offered, the method used in the program is the 'Custody Resolution Method', reporting a combination of coaching and software solutions that provide divorcing families with a resolution to get out of the Court system (Conscious Co-Parenting Institute, 2022). No costs for the program or staff qualifications were supplied.

Also recommended to the Researcher was the "Parental Alienation Study Group, Inc. (PASG)". PASG is an international, not-for-profit corporation with approximately 800 members, primarily mental health and legal professionals, from 62 countries (Parental Alienation Study Group, 2022, p. 1). The Researcher investigated the PASG website for resources pertaining to treatment and interventions for children and adult survivors of PA and SPA. The first blog, under the heading of 'Interventions', mentioned treatments for children experiencing PA but did not mention the severity level (mild, moderate, or severe) of the interventions referred to. The article was by Erel (2022) from Israel, who suggested that PA should be handled as a medical emergency. Erel indicates that children of PA should be triaged and evaluated in Family Court and then moved through an emergency room and on to experts for treatment for recommendations by social workers who have experience with the family (Erel, 2022).

The PASG website also featured a section titled 'Research Supported by PASG', which included a final report titled 'The Clinical and Legal Management of Parental Alienation in the United Kingdom' by Morgan et al. (2020). This report presents the findings of a research project that examines the legal and clinical management of PA in high-conflict separation and divorced families (Morgan et al., 2020). Within the section on therapeutic interventions, the report acknowledged an ongoing debate surrounding PA. However, it specifically mentioned that a comprehensive examination of assessment tools and techniques was beyond the scope of the report (Morgan et al., 2020, p. 40).

Another website, The Family Separation Clinic, focuses on working with children at risk of rejecting a relationship with their loving parent (Family Separation Clinic, 2021). They offer training for MHPs who work with children and families, but no mention is made of training for practitioners who work with adults affected by mild to severe PA. Unfortunately, no details were available regarding the specific

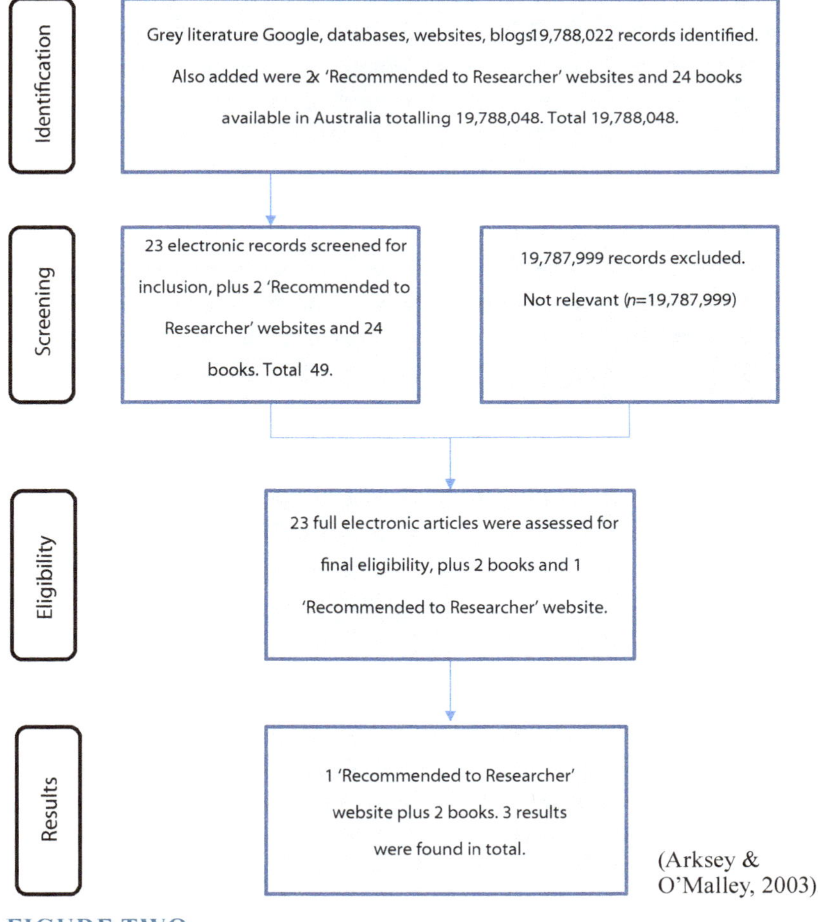

Identification
Grey literature Google, databases, websites, blogs19,788,022 records identified.
Also added were 2x 'Recommended to Researcher' websites and 24 books
available in Australia totalling 19,788,048. Total 19,788,048.
Screening
23 electronic records screened for inclusion, plus 2 'Recommended to Researcher' websites and 24 books. Total 49.
19,787,999 records excluded.
Not relevant (n=19,787,999)
Eligibility
23 full electronic articles were assessed for final eligibility, plus 2 books and 1 'Recommended to Researcher' website.
Results
1 'Recommended to Researcher' website plus 2 books. 3 results were found in total.

(Arksey & O'Malley, 2003).

FIGURE TWO

Results. PRISMA Flowchart of Grey Literature Extended Literature Review

curriculum, protocol, or interventions used and no information about associated costs was reported.

In addition to the aforementioned findings, the Resetting The Family website (Alvarez & Turner, ND) does not offer programs specifically designed for MHPs. Instead, their focus lies on assisting families in creating a new family model through intensive educational programs and employing a case management approach to ensure the family benefits from these programs (Alvarez & Turner, ND). Costs for their services range from $150 to $450 per hour, although the specific country is not specified.

Divorce Study on Adverse Outcomes on Children, Adolescents and Adults

Moving on to a broader perspective, decades of research have yielded studies indicating that parental divorce adversely affects children's outcomes throughout their childhood, adolescence, and adulthood. For example, pioneer researchers Wallerstein and Kelly (1980) wrote and reported on the California Children of Divorce Project in 1971. This research included the initial findings from a five-year post-divorce study from a non-clinical population of 113 children from 60 families aged between two and 18 during their parent's separation (Wallerstein, 1985). PA was not discussed in this study. However, widespread, acute distress was reported from the children when their parents initially broke up, and they requested a universal wish for the family to reconcile and return to an intact family (Wallerstein, 1985).

Within the five-year follow-up, 33% of the children were experiencing moderate to severe depression (Wallerstein, 1985). Preliminary findings also showed that specific psychological effects of divorce could be long-lasting (Wallerstein, 1985). After the initial 5-year study, Wallerstein assumed the responsibility of beginning a further study and conducted a ten-year longitudinal study with the same participants from the earlier research. The motivation behind the ten-year study was due to the concerns expressed by the now adolescents, specifically regarding their ability to establish and sustain a long-lasting, affectionate relationship (Wallerstein, 1985). The adolescents were worried about repeating their parents' divorce in their adult relationships and being frightened by the long dark shadows they had perceived as cast over their parents' divorce. The ten-year study comprised forty young people from 26 families, ranging from 19 to 29, who "regard their parents' divorce as a continuing major influence in their lives" (Wallerstein, 1985, p. 553).

The study reported that many men and women who had participated in the ten-year study seemed troubled and drifting. One-third of the women were wary of commitment and concerned about being betrayed. They reported appearing "caught up in a web of short-lived sexual relationships" (Wallerstein, 1985, p. 553). Study participants firmly fixed on the identity of being a child of divorce reported being continuously burdened by the memories and unfortunate events of their parent's divorce as well as retained sadness, resentment and a "wistful sense of having missed out on the experience of growing up in an intact family" (Wallerstein, 1985, p. 553). Wallerstein and her associates' findings have left a lasting impact on the topic of children of divorce within the research field, even though there were several methodological flaws noted in Wallerstein's research, including the lack of a comparison set and a lack of calculable scales to measure the children's level of difficulties. Despite these limitations, the research remains influential in the field.

Australian Study on Adult Children of PA

In a separate study, survivors of PA shared their experiences regarding PA and their associated mental health issues (Bentley & Matthewson, 2020). The study consisted of ten participants, comprising eight females and two males, whose ages ranged from 26 to 54. Additionally, the study included three participants from the UK, one from Belgium, and one from Germany. While four women were born in Australia, the study did not specify whether the participants identified as white, multicultural, or Aboriginal/Torres Strait Islander individuals.

Within the data collected under the category of 'mental health' in the previously mentioned study, several categories were identified as commonly experienced by survivors of PA. These categories encompass a wide range of challenges, including low self-esteem, substance use, learning and development difficulties, identity-related issues, education and employment challenges, and relationship difficulties (Bentley & Matthewson, 2020). Additional categories include fear of loss, difficulty trusting others, dysfunctional and abusive relationships, struggle to maintain healthy relationships, grief and loss, anger and emotional pain, and feelings of missing out on a childhood (Bentley & Matthewson, 2020).

The study reported that participants discussed various mental health problems such as anxiety, depression, panic attacks, emotion dysregulation, attention problems, posttraumatic stress disorder (PTSD), dissociation, eating disorders, suicidal ideation, and self-harm (Bentley & Matthewson, 2020, p. 8). Participants explained that symptoms from the previous list were more elevated during childhood when the level of alienation was high and reoccurred again during adulthood (Bentley & Matthewson, 2020). Participants also described that they attributed their mental health problems to being alienated from their TP due to the actions and behaviours of the AP (Bentley & Matthewson, 2020). The discussion chapter within the study notes that most participants described their experience of PA as abuse.

The researchers in the study mentioned above did not provide information regarding the severity levels of PA experienced by the participants. The absence of this information in the study highlights the need to acknowledge the complex trauma this important and vulnerable community faces when seeking support from MHPs for SPA in the following topic.

Emergency Help for SPA Symptoms

As previously stated, survivors may present for help regarding their mental and physical health issues relating to SPA. The survivors may present as a hidden population to emergency departments, general practitioners, and mental health practices. Consequently, MHPs may find themselves treating symptoms stemming from SPA abuse, not the SPA itself. For example, the Researcher captured data from the recruitment phase of these studies. An excluded potential study participant (an emergency department mental health nurse) who did not meet the criteria for these studies personally communicated to the Researcher about the survivors presenting at the emergency department where he works. For example, this nurse reported;

> In the emergency department, we see an extensive variety of issues and problems, mostly from people being suicidal and some social disturbance. I would expect we see several people you would define as survivors of severe parental alienation, but that would not be their immediate need. I see survivors of severe parental alienation, but I don't explore the issue deeply in therapy. I don't have any formed opinions or understanding of treatments that can be used in therapy. I wouldn't even know where to start (Name withheld for confidentiality, personal communication, October 16, 2021).

Lack of Professional Knowledge

The previous extract was reflected in the following research reporting that practitioners who work with families and children of SPA can often feel daunted, overwhelmed, and helpless due to a lack of clear published guidelines (Haines et al., 2020). However, no such evidence was discovered during the extended literature review regarding MHPs working with survivors. Considering that practitioners who work with children of SPA feel this way, the Researcher speculated whether practitioners who work with survivors might also feel a similar way. Consequently, these studies' interview questions asked MHPs about this quandary. As a result, the emotional and physical challenges encountered by MHPs when working with children and adults affected by SPA were replicated in these studies in conjunction with additional data that has not been captured previously on this subject. The findings are presented in Volume Two, 'Results, Chapter Six, Mental Health Practitioners'.

Complex Intersecting Traumas of SPA

Previous researchers have emphasised the harmful mechanisms associated with survivors of SPA. However, limited attention has been afforded to the comprehensive range of severe and prolonged physical and psychological CITs suffered by adults who were victims of SPA, leaving MHPs uncertain about how to treat them effectively.

Physical Health

As previously mentioned, adults exposed to severe levels of violence as children can experience symptoms that can manifest into long-term adverse effects (Baker, 2007). For example, adverse physical effects are the number one cause of death in adults who have experienced complex trauma as children (Felitti et al., 1998). This previous research result has been replicated in these studies' results among the survivors and the MHPs.

Mental Health

Adverse psychological effects can present in various academic, physical, psychological, emotional, and social difficulties (Baker, 2007). The challenge practitioners face is a significant concern due to the profound implications on individuals who have endured childhood abuse, maltreatment, and family dysfunction. These individuals have navigated life without the fundamental foundations of secure attachment, encouragement, guidance, and nurturance from primary caregivers.

Consequently, as survivors transition into adulthood, they are burdened with substantial difficulties (Ellis et al., 2019). MHPs must know the wide range of CITs that survivors may present with during a therapeutic session. For example, childhood memories of feeling rejected, unloved, criticised, threatened, subordinate, and alone (Verrocchio et al., 2019). These memories, feelings and experiences can result in internalised uncertainty models about the world and themselves combined with various defensive and submissive behaviours (Verrocchio et al., 2019).

The findings of this review highlight a significant gap in the disparity between the prevalence of mental health and physical consequences experienced by survivors and the limited availability and suitability of treatment options provided by MHPs. Knowledge of the effects and symptoms of SPA and the neurobiological impact on survivors is crucial so that the MHP can begin to engage and respond without causing further harm to the survivor. Previous research emphasises that effective PA therapy necessitates practitioners to comprehensively understand the specific issues they are addressing (Baker, 2006). For example, survivors may exhibit various symptoms that encompass behavioural impairments such as extreme hostility, defiance, withdrawal, and disobedience. Additionally, emotional impairments can manifest as open contempt and a lack of genuine love, appreciation, or affection. Furthermore, cognitive impairments may exist (Gardner, 1998; Kelly, 2010).

Current Treatment for PA and SPA

Thousands of mental health and legal professionals who work with divorcing families have recognised PA as a phenomenon (Verrocchio et al., 2019). Thousands are also treating the symptoms of PA, such as psychiatrists, psychologists, social workers, and family counsellors (Verrocchio et al., 2019). These studies aim to support survivors in their healing process by empowering them to express their thoughts and uncover 'hidden truths'. These 'hidden truths' may have been suppressed, inaccessible, misunderstood, distorted, or ignored (Bergen, 1993) concerning their symptoms and subsequent treatment experiences.

Conclusion

This extended literature review has reported on the gap in research related to the lack of treatment protocols and understanding of SPA in mental health practice within the peer-reviewed and grey literature and emphasised the importance of developing specialised knowledge among MHPs to support this vulnerable population effectively. Additionally, the chapter highlighted the adverse outcomes associated with divorce, PA, and SPA, particularly the impact on children. Given the scarcity of peer-reviewed literature explicitly focused on these topics, MHPs must approach the subject carefully and discerningly while avoiding unwarranted assumptions.

Additionally, given the limited research in this area, it is advisable to exercise caution and refrain from making overly definitive claims when working with SPA survivors. Rather than overstating any current understanding, adopting a balanced approach developed from empathy and curiosity is vital. This careful strategy will entail drawing upon the existing knowledge while acknowledging the research limitations and the need to explore adult trauma further. By adopting such an approach, we can navigate the current gaps in the literature and strive for a deeper understanding of SPA, paving the way for future advancements and research in this burgeoning field.

The findings of this extended literature review indicate the necessity for MHPs to acquire a higher level of professional development to comprehend the complex dynamics involving the biological, psychological, familial, and social factors that contribute to the intergenerational cycles of trauma and violence in the context of SPA.

Furthermore, the study emphasises the significance of incorporating the concept of ACEs and recognising the presence of complex intersecting traumas (CITs) when providing therapeutic support to survivors.

As a result, this review strongly supports the development of a comprehensive treatment protocol for MHPs that incorporates both behavioural and relational interventions. Such a protocol should specifically target instances of maltreatment and abuse within the context of SPA, aiming to address and mitigate the risk of recurrent victimisation for survivors.

Chapter Four

Foundations of Methodology: A Comprehensive Overview for Both PhD Studies

This chapter describes a detailed explanation of the procedures and methods employed in these studies to address the main research question and the sub-questions for the two cohorts—namely, survivors and the MHPs who work with them therapeutically. In presenting the twin study PhD across both volumes, the researcher aims to ensure consistency and accessibility of information for both MHPs and adult survivors. Throughout both volumes, the researcher will include the same methodology sections that detail how the research was conducted, ensuring transparency and clarity for all readers. These methodology sections will offer insights into the approaches, techniques, and considerations relevant to both MHPs and adult survivors. By including this information in both volumes, the researcher seeks to empower both audiences with a comprehensive understanding of the research process and its implications for their respective roles and experiences.

As these studies have reported, childhood exposure to severe PABs can have enduring adverse effects on survivors. However, MHPs often lack the necessary training and knowledge to support these survivors effectively. The challenges are amplified by the scarcity of professional development opportunities and the absence of established best-practice treatment protocols for practitioners to reference. To bridge the knowledge gap, the Researcher chose a qualitative approach. This choice was motivated by the limited availability of data from previous studies on SPA identified in the extended literature review. Merriam and Tisdell (2016) argue that research focusing on understanding the perspectives of those being studied can significantly impact people's lives.

This chapter will present the methodology in two sections: the methodological positioning and the research design. Within qualitative research, it is important to recognise and articulate the philosophical beliefs that underlie the research (Cresswell & Poth, 2017). It also offers a more natural and holistic method of inquiry, allowing for a deeper understanding of the phenomena by gathering rich and nuanced data for collection and analysis (Cresswell & Poth, 2017).

The Researcher chose qualitative research as it encompasses a range of traditions and approaches that prioritise the study participants' perspective over the researcher's (Boswell & Babchuk, 2022). Choosing a qualitative route for the research was also due to the Researcher intuitively knowing that many things she sees in session cannot be rationally measured or quantified (Finlay, 2011). Qualitative research also enables the practitioner's views, theories, intuitive hunches, and approaches to be shared, allowing other practitioners to draw from their experience (Finlay, 2011).

According to Finlay (2011, p.5), MHPs argue that quantitative measures do not inherently capture the values of practitioners or inform their practice. In contrast, practitioners' interests extend beyond mere simplistic behavioural evaluations as they seek a more comprehensive understanding of their field (Finlay, 2011). In this regard, qualitative research emerges as a more plausible and practical approach, offering an additional, suitable solution to address their broader concerns (Finlay, 2011, p. 5). In this context, qualitative research is posited as a more harmonious and practical approach offering the potential to address the broader concerns of MHPs while providing a more profound, extended scope of the investigation into the complexity of therapeutic practice.

Philosophical Orientation

The decisions made in research, including establishing objectives and the outcomes sought, are greatly influenced by philosophical orientations (Moon & Blackman, 2017). Likewise, these orientations are crucial in shaping the study's direction and framework in qualitative research. Four key orientations have been identified as particularly impactful (Moon & Blackman, 2017):

Of note, the Researcher believes that ontology, which pertains to the nature of reality and the claims made about knowledge, is intricately connected to utilising qualitative research methods. These methods serve as a valuable guide, allowing the Researcher to investigate and comprehend the complex and multifaceted perspectives of study participants. In this context, ontology refers to the researcher's understanding of the nature of reality and the claims they make pertaining to knowledge. It encompasses questions about the essence and existence of the phenomenon under investigation. For example, what claims to truth can researchers make about reality? (Moon & Blackman, 2017).

Epistemology

The assumptions of social constructionism form the epistemological foundation for these studies. A social constructionist epistemology standpoint also guided the thematic analysis, as SPA is a sociocultural issue influenced by socially and professionally constructed norms. Epistemology studies show how individuals acquire knowledge and validate their claims, shedding light on researchers' understanding of knowledge acquisition (Moon & Blackman, 2017). It also involves investigating how researchers gain knowledge about the subject of their inquiry and the criteria they use to establish the reliability of their findings (Moon & Blackman, 2017). Finally, the researcher can also explore epistemology and its influence on the research design by examining the relationship between an object and a subject (Moon & Blackman, 2017).

Axiology

On the other hand, Axiology focuses on the role of values within the research process, particularly the impact of importance within the relationship between methodology and methods. It requires researchers to acknowledge and consider their personal and cultural values, including biases, assumptions, roles in the research process, preferences, and how these may impact the study (Zareen & Larsen, 2018). These values allow researchers to acknowledge the importance of recording biases, cultural and personal values, preferences, assumptions and how they influence the study. Researchers must be committed to addressing and adhering to these factors to ensure the validity and integrity of the research (Zareen & Larsen, 2018).

Social Constructionism

Social constructionism refers to societal influences shaping our perception of reality (Galbin, 2014). It is a theory in sociology that explores how we collectively create and interpret the world around us through communication and interaction (Galbin, 2014). Social constructionists recognise the social nature of human beings while encouraging individuals to share their own stories (Galbin, 2014). Social constructionism believes that even though social and inherited factors exist simultaneously, it does not deny any influence on genetic heritage but instead chooses to study the social influences within the community and individual life (Galbin, 2014).

The core premise of social constructionism maintains that human experience is shaped by historical, cultural, and linguistic factors and that individuals actively negotiate meanings (Willig, 2001). Thus, the central research objective is to identify and comprehend the diverse methods employed by a culture to construct social reality (Willig, 2001). Social constructionism also presents a comprehensive framework for investigating the process of meaning-making. Social constructionism posits that everyday phenomena are constructed through language (Willig, 2001). This theory is guided by the fundamental social constructionist principle that human experience is historically, culturally, and linguistically mediated and that people actively negotiate meanings (Willig, 2001).

Furthermore, social constructionist research aims to identify and comprehend a culture's diverse means of constructing social reality (Willig, 2001). The complexity of social reality demands a multifaceted and layered approach to inquiry (Willig, 2001). By employing a theoretical framework and suitable methodologies, researchers can gain insights into meaning-making's multidimensional and dynamic nature, shedding light on how individuals derive significance, construct individual narratives, and navigate their personal experiences within a larger sociocultural context (Willig, 2001).

According to Burr (1995), social constructionism emerged within the intellectual and cultural postmodern movement. It challenges the idea that there is an ultimate truth in the world that results from concealed structures, such as hidden psychic constructions that account for the psychological phenomenon (Schultheiss & Wallace, 2012). This concept contrasted with the Western modernist tradition that emphasised the idea of a self-contained person with measurable traits (Schultheiss & Wallace, 2012).

Furthermore, social constructionism has distinguishing identifying marks that reject any assumption proposed regarding the nature of the mind and causality theories (Galbin, 2014). For example, it emphasises the interrelatedness and complexity of the many dimensions to the individuals within communities, including challenging the majority of common-sense knowledge we apply to ourselves and the surrounding world (Galbin, 2014).

Berger and Luckmann (1991) report that socialisation occurs through contact and language with significant others who mediate the objective realities within society, give it meaning and send it on its way, which is then internalised by the first individual (Andrews 2012). Berger and

Luckmann (1991) suggest that maintaining a conversation is the best way to sustain, modify and reconstruct one's subjective reality (Andrews, 2012). Berger and Luckmann also suggest that dialogue nourishes and reconstructs subjective reality (Andrews, 2012). For example, shared concepts assume a reality taken for granted, such as "have a great day" (Andrews, 2012).

Relativist Lens

Additionally, social constructionism within psychology is an overarching title for an expanding group of alternative approaches working to understand the human experience (Harper, 2008). Social constructionism mainly concerns how knowledge is constructed and assumes that knowledge occurs in the social processes between humans (Harper, 2008). Within the differing variations of social constructionism, the familiar relativism-realism debates concerning the position afforded to truth and reality continue (Liebrucks, 2001). Arguments have previously focused on how humans prefer one perception of the world over another, especially when the 'reality' is thought to be inaccessible within the ontology of relativism (Liebrucks, 2001). Through adopting a relativist lens, these studies explore the nuanced perspectives and complex meanings constructed within the data while aiming to capture the rich tapestry within the subjective realities. These studies also seek to move beyond the limitations of a singular truth and embrace the complex interpretations and understandings within a relativist framework. These studies employed a social constructionist framework guided by a sensitive research method proposed by Liamputtong (2019). This approach was chosen because some participants in both study cohorts identified themselves as having lived experience before and during the interviews.

Sensitive Research Approach

The Researcher carefully noted the literature on vulnerable people and acknowledged the complex nature of their experiences, including behavioural and emotional impairments. A 'sensitive research methods' approach was adopted to address these concerns, as advocated by Liamputtong (2019). This approach emphasises the necessity for specific considerations, utmost care, and enhanced protection when working with vulnerable populations. As Shivayogi (2013, p. 53) describes, vulnerable people are the disadvantaged sub-segment of the community that requires meticulous attention, specific ancillary considerations, and augmented protections in research.

Heeding this description, Liamputtong (2019) points out that performing research with participants deemed vulnerable and marginalised can present researchers with unique and valuable opportunities, and this theme is shown in many chapters within her research. However, Shivayogi (2019) identifies the absence of uniformity or standards in monitoring and evaluating quantum risks for biomedical research for vulnerable populations. This lack of safeguards inhibits stakeholders' understanding and evaluation in this field (Shivayogi, 2013). The Researcher came to appreciate the importance of this layer to the research methodology due to the parallel with professional practice relating to the client's trauma experiences.

Contemporary Trauma Theory

Consequently, adopting contemporary trauma theory (CTT) as the foundation for trauma-informed care (TIC) within social work and co-occurring trauma (Goodman, 2017) becomes crucial in ensuring informed and comprehensive approaches to address trauma-related issues. The development of CTT represents a shift within professional practice regarding how mental health professionals perceive and treat trauma survivors (Goodman, 2017). By adopting the lens of TIC, MHPs recognise that poor clinical presentations and maladaptive functioning observed in clients can stem from unresolved trauma and diminished self-regulatory skills (Goodman, 2017). This understanding allows MHPs to provide more compassionate and empathic support to clients as they navigate their trauma. By acknowledging and recognising the role of trauma, MHPs can create a safe and understanding therapeutic environment promoting healing and growth. Conversely, when MHPs disregard the role of trauma within the clinical population, this decision may lead to an inaccurate diagnosis and subsequent unhelpful treatment, which may result in higher attrition rates or even a relapse back into trauma for clients (Goodman, 2017).

According to Alexander (2015), broadening the focus on trauma or maltreatment may assist in discontinuing the cycles of violence. This idea includes developing protective factors and resilience, which creates pathways to higher levels of these aspects, including any existing positive relationships that offer emotional support (Alexander, 2015). These factors can come from a loved one or psychotherapist and can help to modify the effects of previously abusive relationships (DuMont et al., 2007; Egeland et al., 1988). A key question for MHPs to consider is, "How does an individual with a history of maltreatment and trauma escape this cycle to become a loving parent and partner?" (Alexander, 2015, p. 13). This question can be answered differently based on which conceptual model is used.

Methodology

The following research design describes the procedures and methods employed by these two studies to explore the perspectives of MHPs who work with survivors and the survivors themselves. The qualitative methods used to gather data from these cohorts were achieved using a semi-structured interview style. Please refer to Appendices Six and Seven for the questions used in the semi-structured interviews. According to an older reference (Burr, 2003), this approach has become more popular over recent years due to the idea that the generating of theory and analysis is shaped by the researcher's dealings with the world and cultural influences, which can then impact their interpretations of the gathered data.

In order to gain insights into the experiences and perspectives of survivors of SPA and the MHPs who support them, the study examined two distinct cohorts comprising a total of twenty-one participants. Eleven survivors (who accessed MHPs for SPA symptoms) and ten MHPs consulted with and offered treatment to survivors in their practice (either face-to-face or via a computer). Participants were recruited locally and internationally through worldwide social media platforms such as Facebook, LinkedIn, and international PA research (The Parental Alienation Study Group, 'PASG') and PA-specific support groups. Locally, participants were recruited through community mental health agency networks across Australia.

In addition, a snowball sample was adopted to recruit participants. Snowball sampling involves asking a participant in the research to recommend other research conversation participants and is used to access hard-to-reach groups where a frame for sampling does not exist or a researcher cannot access this particular group (Walter, 2019). Further recruiting included liaising with MHPs from universities and agencies interested in the study.

To recruit participants, the Researcher posted an Expression of Interest flyer (please refer to Appendix Eight, Volume Two) to social media sites asking specific questions to survivors. The Researcher then posted a second Expression of Interest Flyer to social media sites asking specific questions to MHPs who treat survivors (please refer to Appendix Nine, Volume Two). Interested participants who contacted the Researcher by email to obtain more information about the study were sent the following inclusion criteria to view and respond to;

Participants were prepared and informed of what the study expected from them (Finlay, 2011). Once the Researcher determined who met the criteria outlined in the flyer, the Researcher sent the applicable qualifying information to the next applicant in line, and they were asked to fill in the forms and send them back. Information received from potential study participants who did not meet the criteria in their applications via email was handled with utmost confidentiality and in compliance with ethical guidelines. In these cases, the Researcher ensured that the email containing the application was stored securely. The email was not shared with anyone who was not directly involved in these studies.

Additionally, the Researcher promptly informed the participants within 24 hours that they did not meet the criteria for inclusion in these studies while assuring them that their information would be handled confidentially and not be used for any other purpose. This selection process was based on 'first in, first serve' criteria and not selected randomly or cherry-picked. Choosing study participants on this basis was considered important to maintain a clear, unbiased data sample.

To meet the inclusion criteria, survivors were required to:

1. Identify as having been exposed to SPA as children.
2. Have reunited with their targeted parent.
3. Have received traditional therapeutic treatment for SPA from a mental health practitioner with a bachelor's level or post-graduate qualification.
4. Be over the age of 21 years.
5. Not be currently experiencing acute symptoms or significant stress or crisis.

To meet the inclusion criteria, MHPs who treat adult survivors were required to:

1. Be treating or have treated adult survivors of SPA.
2. Hold a minimum level of a bachelor's degree or post-graduate qualification.

Reflexivity

Research reflexivity involves acknowledging the power dynamics and hierarchical relationships between the researcher and study participant, as Raheim et al. (2016) described. This acknowledgement signifies a commitment to establishing an anti-authoritarian relationship where the researcher is conscious of their position and its influence on the research process. This includes examining who conducts the research, the underlying research agenda, and how the experiences of both 'superior' and 'inferior' knowledge positions intersect during data collection. By engaging in reflexivity, the researcher strives to create a more equitable and inclusive research environment that respects the perspectives and voices of all participants involved (Raheim et al., 2016).

Reflexivity, a widely embraced practice in qualitative research, prompts researchers to engage in critical self-reflection, actively considering their position within the research process and the broader social context in which their work takes place (Linabary et al., 2020). For example, feminist researchers advocate for reflexivity as a comprehensive and holistic process that extends throughout the researcher's journey (Hesse-Bibber & Piatelli, 2012). These authors contend that embracing reflexivity reminds researchers to ask transformative and diverse questions while fostering relationships with study participants, creating more inclusive, alternative representations (Hesse-Bibber & Piatelli, 2012). To address concerns about the power dynamics inherent in the researcher-participant relationship, feminist reflexive approaches have emerged as a response. By engaging in reflexivity, researchers aim to critically examine and challenge their own assumptions, biases, and positions of privilege while striving for a more equitable research process. These approaches, such as those advocated by Wilkinson (1988) and Reinharz (1992), aim to shift the balance of power towards participants (Wilkinson, 1988; Reinharz, 1992).

Bias

Other researchers, such as Hertz (1997), emphasise the importance of researcher self-awareness and explicit positioning within research, arguing that researchers are subject to various influences throughout the research process (Hertz, 1997). These influences impact the research questions, the subjects studied, and the representation and writing of findings (Hertz, 1997). Reflexivity enables researchers to identify and mitigate potential biases, leading to more accurate accounts of the social world (Hertz, 1997). For example, confirmation bias may occur when researchers seek out or give importance to evidence that aligns with their existing views or experiences, resulting in selective observation, undervaluing, or overlooking evidence contrary to their beliefs (National School of Healthcare Science, n.d.).

Within this section, the Researcher provides an account of their role, their choices, and how the data was co-produced following their interpretations. By choosing to write this, the Researcher acknowledges that her role in gathering and coding data has not been through the eyes of a neutral observer (Silverman, 1997). Decisions regarding approaching the research require the researcher to be responsible and accountable for their decisions and actions. Willig (2013) reports that researchers have the potential to shape and influence research personally and as a theorist and a thinker. The concepts are defined as personal reflexivity (referring to the person) and epistemological reflexivity (referring to the theorist/thinker). This allows the researcher to acknowledge their identity, biases, and theoretical and epistemological views. Also included are the interests and personal values that the Researcher has held and the elaboration of any expectations that impact the co-production of the data and analysis process (Cromby, 1999). This encompasses the Researcher's own lived experience, her role as a practitioner-researcher and her interest in developing a treatment protocol for survivors.

Reflexivity was acknowledged by the Researcher as a necessary instrument to address her positionality and was documented using a reflection journal. Research reflexivity is different to reflexivity that is practised professionally by MHPs. Professional reflexivity is described as drawing on the practitioners' heartfelt wisdom and subtle body changes that allow clients insight into their personal experiences (Finlay, 2011). Reflexivity allows the practitioner's body to act as a type of somatic compass (Milloy, 2010). Finlay (2011) argues that reflexivity needs to be applied to the participant and researcher due to its importance in research.

During the research, the Researcher realised that she had numerous assumptions as a clinical psychotherapist that warranted a timely reflexivity pause (Blakely, 2022). During these pauses, the Researcher needed to properly consider the sensitive topic she was exploring beyond the initial interview process. Within the pause, the Researcher reflected upon being a "practitioner-researcher with a critical gaze" (Blakely, 2022, p. 6) and combined this view with a sensitive research approach to capture the personal perspectives of study participants with lived experience.

Furthermore, in conducting and carrying out the research, the Researcher became aware of several factors that influenced the analysis. First, the Researcher was aware of her personal reasons for engaging in a study for survivors borne out of her own experience as an adult survivor of SPA who has never been able to find a practitioner who knew how to work with her or provide treatment options. Due to this, the Researcher has chosen to find the answers for herself through these studies.

The Researcher's personal reasons and past experiences as an adult survivor of SPA can potentially introduce bias into the research process. To mitigate confirmation bias, the Researcher remained vigilant and adopted strategies to minimise its impact. This included being transparent about her personal background and motivations in the research report, employing rigorous research methodologies, employing independent coders or reviewers for data analysis, and actively seeking and considering diverse perspectives and contrary evidence.

Throughout the data collection phase, interviews were recorded from sessions on Zoom, which were uploaded into NVivo and transcribed and printed onto pages and reread through a reflexive lens. Any questions or challenging content were documented at the time and spoken about during supervisory meetings if required. Reflections were pondered upon during the Researcher's quieter times. Any biases the Researcher felt were documented and brought to the primary supervisor for discussion. For example, personal interests and ethical considerations issues arising from the study. In addition, as part of her Master's degree program, the Researcher actively engaged in two years of in-depth discussions focused on identifying and addressing biases within advanced research skills. This extensive training was crucial in equipping the Researcher with the necessary knowledge and skills to recognise and mitigate biases effectively.

Data Collection Method and Process

During the development stage of the interview process and after the extended literature review, the Researcher collaborated with a clinical psychologist who possessed expert knowledge in the SPA area. Together, they formed a semi-structured interview schedule that addressed the research question, the sub-questions, and the study's aims. The questions were centred around reviewing existing published literature while noting any perceived gaps in the research and maintaining an exploratory nature, which led to the development of questions.

These studies utilised a semi-structured interviewing style, recognised as effective for investigating social enquiry (Charmaz, 2014). The application of semi-structured interviews in these studies followed an intensive and comprehensive method that allowed for capturing the perspectives of the two study cohorts. The semi-structured interviews consisted of non-directive, open-ended questions formulated to produce rich, quality data. Semi-structured interviews establish rapport with the participants and explore secondary subject matter areas stemming from their life experiences while informing their introspective interpretation of the phenomenon (Lauterbach, 2018). Within the semi-structured interview protocol, specific questions are designed before the interview, and every specific question may not be asked; however, all the topics are covered (Lauterbach, 2018). Semi-structured interviews include non-directive, open-ended questions designed to stimulate quality data (Lauterbach, 2018). Peavey's (1990) 'Art of Strategic Questioning' was used to design the questions in the study and analyse the data collected on the experiences of the survivors and the MHPs.

Lastly, it is important to note that whilst qualitative research and the employment of thematic analysis aims to advantage 'true' individualised, subjective knowledge, this notion seems to be a goal rather than reality. During this thesis, the Researcher has tried to stay aware of her shifting biases and lived experience expectations while reflecting intermittently on how this influences the findings.

Throughout history, scholars have described qualitative research as creating new knowledge without prearranged responses and critically evaluating and understanding people's perspectives and complex concepts (Creswell & Poth, 2017; Denzin & Lincoln, 2000; Fine et al., 2000). To ensure a complete understanding of the SPA phenomenon, the Researcher gathered data from two distinct cohorts: survivors who could provide new insights and perspectives based on their personal experiences and MHPs who possessed the expertise and worked with this client group (van Manen, 1990). By including both groups, the Researcher aimed to collect "good data" (Cresswell & Poth, 2017, p. 148) that was information-rich, purposefully sampled and could be compared and cross-matched for further research to be developed.

Participant Interviews

Most participants' interviews lasted approximately 60 to 90 minutes, but some survivor interviews went longer. The survivor research interviews took longer than initially anticipated, and the Researcher felt that she needed more empathy and sensitivity to obtain as complete a description as possible regarding the participant's experience (Giorgi, 2009, p. 122). Participants were constantly monitored and observed for signs of emotional distress. According to the participant's presentation, the interviews changed from a formal focus to an informal focus during the process. For example, some survivors experienced differing emotional states, requiring more time and a calmer approach.

One survivor participant reported that their emotional distress was due to having never spoken about their SPA trauma before and felt safe enough to speak knowing that the Researcher was also an adult survivor herself. For example, previous research reports that therapist self-disclosure is crucial in fostering a robust alliance between therapists and their clients (Cleary & Armour, 2022). By sharing personal experiences, therapists can create a sense of solidarity with their clients, especially when they have lived through similar situations themselves (Cleary & Armour, 2022). This mutual understanding can lead to a stronger therapeutic relationship and better outcomes for the client (Cleary & Armour, 2022).

Due to the emotionality of the interviews, the Researcher presupposes that some survivors may not remember everything they said. During the interviews, the Researcher noted that it was the first time that some of the survivor research participants had spoken about their long-lived experiences of severe childhood trauma. For example, the survivors explained their perspectives regarding attending sessions with MHPs to talk about their childhood abuse as context, and these examples became part of their negative and positive perspectives relating to the study questions. Due to this, the interviews were immediately handled more delicately, and the allocated times were adapted to a slower style than originally anticipated.

The additional time was reported to the Higher Degree by Research Coordinator and the ethics department at USC as soon as this previously flagged potential factor emerged in the data. The USC ethics department granted extra time for interviews once this foreseen circumstance appeared within this vulnerable cohort. This change in the research regarding interviews taking longer than initially anticipated and needing more empathy and sensitivity to obtain as complete a description as possible regarding the experience the participant has lived through has been reported in previous research (Giorgi, 2009, p.122). Consequently, more data was collected, reflected in the transcribed pages. Researcher notes and the coding were printed out before the thematic analysis began.

However, due to the complexity and sensitivity of their experiences, the survivors often required additional time during the interviews, creating a noticeable contrast with the efficient, confident and concise responses provided by the MHPs. During the interview and observation process, the Researcher wrote notes and reflected them to the study participant with empathy and compassion for accuracy. Guiding questions, reflections and prompts were elicited (Finlay, 2011). Interviews with this cohort progressed with spontaneity and fluidity, allowing the Researcher to ask questions as required. Also, unlike the adult survivor cohort, none of the MHPs showed signs of emotional distress or reported needing extra support while discussing their SPA perspectives.

Thematic Analysis of Data

Given the exploratory nature of the current study, thematic analysis emerged as a valuable method for capturing the perspectives of the research participants while uncovering variations and commonalities in their perspectives (Braun & Clarke, 2006; King, 2004). By utilising thematic analysis, the Researcher was able to synthesise the key elements within the data, resulting in the formulation of a comprehensive set of results (Nowell et al., 2017). This methodological choice provided a systematic means to identify and examine recurrent themes while offering the opportunity to capture the complexities and nuances within the participants' narratives. Employing thematic analysis provides an opportunity to build upon existing knowledge about the needs and experiences of survivors and offers an opportunity to discover unexpected and under-researched concepts.

Data Management

Data storage and management will follow the USC policy guideline 36, "ethical issues in using the audio-visual recording in human research", which states that data collected will be stored on a password-protected computer and in a locked filing cabinet when not required. Altogether, twenty interviews were undertaken and transcribed verbatim. These transcripts yielded over 340 pages of data from the survivors and approximately 250 pages of data from the MHPs. The interviews for the survivors and the MHPs were conducted in the same time frame between February 2022 and April 2022. Transcribed interviews were notated shortly after being conducted to capture as much accurate detail as possible before the recollection of the interview diminished within the Researcher's memory. In addition, any unanticipated themes identified early within the interview process were observed and incorporated into any following interviews, refining the interview schedule.

Similarly, themes that the Researcher initially thought would be important but weren't elaborated on or identified by the research participants were gradually removed from the data. Data collection was continually revised according to the interpretation of the smaller units of meaning based on the Researcher's current interpretations of the larger units of meaning. This, in turn, led to new and improved interpretations of the larger units of meaning themselves. This process was repeated slowly and consciously, which improved the interpretation using circular movements.

By reflecting on the perspectives of both cohorts, the Researcher increased the personal perspectives, which improved the interpretation as a whole. By reflecting on the perspectives, the understanding of participants' perspectives increased. The Researcher continued to move back and forth between the data and different levels of analysis while interpreting the context concerning its elements in terms of their context.

Coding

Coding is how factual and detailed information gathered from the research is analysed and transformed into more theoretical concepts (Boyatziz, 1998; Bryant & Charmaz, 2007). Four main phases of coding were conducted: 1. 'open coding', where the Researcher coded every line systematically; 2. 'selective coding', where the more detailed categories were analysed and conceptualised; 3. 'focused coding', which used the earlier defined codes and applied them to add large amounts of data; and 4. 'axial coding', where relationships between the categories and subcategories were investigated and developed (Charmaz, 2014). The emerging themes and sub-themes informed the Researcher as they read and reread the coded research participant information. Continual comparative analysis systematically and thoroughly identified similarities and variations that enhanced the researcher's understanding and knowledge (Boyatziz, 1998; Bryant & Charmaz, 2007). One example included research participants from both populations reporting a lack of education about SPA and its effect on the community. Near the conclusion of the interviewing process, it became clear that survivors and professionals identified shared themes and concerns. Please see Chapters Five and Six, Volume Two, for the results.

The following framework outlined in Table One was used to arrange and record the data analysis. The table is a sample from the survivors and MHP interviews, including the original transcripts, exploratory comments, emerging themes and main themes. The purpose of the data analysis was twofold: to reveal underlying concepts and establish specific experiences while ensuring that these findings accurately reflected the individual experiences of the research participants.

TABLE ONE

Extract from Adult Survivor and MHP Interview Transcripts

Page 1	Step One: Original transcript adult survivor of SPA	Step Two: Exploratory comments	Step Three: Emerging Themes	Step Four: Main Themes
	There's not enough education, there's not enough help, and I feel like the only person that can really help me is myself, unfortunately, and sometimes I don't know how to do that because I'm grieving.	Awareness and identification of a lack of knowledge among practitioners. Complete reliance on self for help. Identification of lifelong grief over SPA experiences. Vulnerable. Concerned. High emotional impact. Internal turmoil. Loss of hope concerning a recovery.	Unable to find good professional help due to a lack of training. Feelings of despair, hopelessness, and confusion. Identification of somatic symptoms. Identification of personal lack of understanding of PA education.	The identification of adult survivor presenting mental and physical health symptoms by practitioners need further research, development and training regarding clinical diagnosis and treatment. The development of psychoeducation for adult survivors, especially around lifelong grief. Creation of an expanded worldview of PA treatment protocols.
Page 2	**Step One: Original transcript MHP**	**Step Two: Exploratory comments**	**Step Three: Emerging Themes**	**Step Four: Main Themes**
	I don't think a lot of practitioners work with adult survivors very often.	Unknown factors within their professional community.	Identification of a lack of professional development and support for practitioners in the PA field.	Statistics on survivor presentation skills require more research.
	So, it's a bit of a niche area that we step into.	Identification of the uniqueness and specialty knowledge required when working in the SPA field.	Identification of a challenging context. Potential isolation. Emotional impact. A lack of professional development among practitioners.	More research into the needs of MHPs, including vicarious trauma impacts. The identification of adult survivor symptoms by practitioners needs further research, development, and training regarding clinical diagnosis.

	I'm curious about that. I wonder if they are working with survivors, and they just don't know it.	Curious, concerned, reflective. Professional knowledge of other practitioners working with SPA is a concern.	Developing insights into MHPs' roles within SPA	Creation of an expanded world view on SPA treatment protocols.

Data from the survivors were rigorously and systematically analysed according to thematic analysis first, and then data from the MHPs was analysed using the same method. This was achieved by the Researcher reading through and highlighting important sections relevant to the research questions. From the initial coding in NVivo, the first round of raw data was reread. The Researcher looked for lines that participants may have said were not captured in the first sweep. The Researcher decided to capture and incorporate these into the findings even if they were not a dominant theme in case they led to something more interesting later. The Researcher tried to capture all angles and nuances of what participants from both groups had stated in their experiences. The initial round was used to identify core themes upon which to build. While looking further over the data, the Researcher explored the similarities and relationships between the chunks of data and moved toward considering developing them into themes. Once the themes emerged, they were returned to the raw data to confirm their existence. This was performed repeatedly until the Researcher felt that saturation had occurred.

To add rigour, objectivity, and reliability to the transcript data, three other PhD researchers blindly scored a random mix of uncoded transcripts from both cohorts to read code and highlight. They were encouraged to write notes in the margins if anything came to mind. When this was complete, the transcripts were then returned to the Researcher. None of the analysts had a personal relationship with any participants, and no conflict of interest was declared. The trustworthiness and credibility of the data analysis were improved because of these factors.

The second round of data analysis was performed to identify sub-themes or themes that the Researcher thought existed but may not have garnered the support needed to turn into a theme as initially thought. During this important time, the Researcher was mindful about reflecting on how to capture and demonstrate that she had systematically and methodically analysed the data while thoughtfully and considerately reflecting on what the research participants had said. Finally, strong, emergent themes were identified. Quotes by the research participants were then converted into thematic interpretations (Boyatzis, 1998; Charmaz, 2006).

Ethics

The primary focal point for the Researcher was to remember that the study participants involved in the research were individuals with unique experiences, some of whom had never discussed their SPA experiences before. During the study, the dignity of everyone was maintained, regardless of the research or any outcomes. The Researcher was mindful to treat the participants with the highest regard (Salkind, 1991, p. 37) and respect. The research was conducted to minimise distress for the participants and considered the implications of discussion or discovery of potentially criminal behaviour or criminal acts. Furthermore, it is important to clarify that the Researcher did not assume the role of a therapist or counsellor for any research participants (Collins-Mrakas, 2004).

The Researcher applied for and was granted ethics approval with the University of the Sunshine Coast to follow appropriate scientific protocol. The Researcher did not engage in recruiting research participants for interviews until receiving ethics approval. The Researcher obtained ethical clearance from the National Health and Medical Research Council (NHMRC) through the Human Research Ethics Application (HREA), approval number S211642. Participants' welfare, safety, and dignity in these studies were imperative. Participants were treated fairly and equally, not as a means to an end. Therefore, ethical issues were absent during data collection regarding participants and did not influence the research (Collins-Mrakas, 2004).

Participants' social, physical, and psychological well-being was not negatively affected by their participation as far as the Researcher knew from the feedback she was given at the end of the interview. For example, at the end of the interview, the Researcher enquired about how the participants were feeling and if they required any extra support, as a trained counsellor was on standby during and after the interviews. However, they were not requested.

Participants have been protected from physical or psychological harm to the best of the Researcher's ability. None of the participants from the two research cohorts requested a debriefing. Consequently, the Researcher assumed nothing was noted as 'too upsetting' during the research. Additionally, before and after the interviews, all participants were advised to contact Beyond Blue, Lifeline, or their General Practitioner for support as needed. However, the German translator who was employed for one of the survivors did become upset due to the level of child abuse that she had to interpret during the interview. Still, she did not want to access the counselling offer after the interview.

The Researcher also noted that some MHPs expressed feeling worried about potential threats from colleagues who are known as 'experts' in the SPA field due to the information they were offering for these studies. As such, the data has been deidentified to a deeper level to protect their privacy. For example, in the more contentious extracts, names were not mentioned. Instead, these MHPs were listed as anonymous. A further step was removing the ages and sexes of the MHP participants and the organisations they worked with. Please see 'Perspectives of Working with Other Practitioners in the SPA Field-Accounts of Bullying Among PA Professionals' on page 219 for more information.

All participants were informed of the objective of these studies and the design features. The benefits and risks were also explained to the participants by emailing out appropriate information to let them know about the interview and their levels of participation. The research participants' welfare, rights and dignity needed to precede the research requirements. The confidentiality of the participants was assured and conveyed to them before starting. This level of confidentiality was continued by the researchers carrying out the blind interviews, as they were only provided with the pseudonyms of the participants. Consequently, the research was conducted with empathy and non-judgement while creating a safe and supportive environment for study participants to share their perspectives.

Additionally, the Researcher recognised and considered participant diversity, considering gender, ethnicity, and cultural and linguistic diversity. This was undertaken as the Researcher is professionally trained to recognise and respect participants from a CALD background due to her professional training and working in the western suburbs of Sydney for the past 20 years.

In addition, the Researcher has not invaded any participant's private space to collect data without permission from the participants. Participants were not forced to participate at any time. Participants were free to agree to join the research or not for any reason. The participants read, signed, and completed all informed consent forms before the research began. Anything learned about the participant during the research is being held in confidence and securely stored in a locked cabinet at the University of the Sunshine Coast for a minimum of five years, in accordance with the guidelines provided by the NHMRC and the USC ethics department.

Furthermore, should the data be used for the pilot study of a clinical trial, it will be retained accordingly. Study participants have given their consent to use their information in a future clinical trial to develop a treatment protocol. However, if the data is not needed for future studies, it will be adequately shredded to ensure data protection and confidentiality.

Conclusion

In conclusion, this research has encompassed a broad range of important components. This chapter began with adopting a qualitative research approach followed by methodological considerations, including research design, recruitment of the study population, and selection criteria for participants. Appropriate steps were taken to manage bias and promote reflexivity throughout the process. The development of the interview schedule, data collection and thematic analysis played important roles in allowing for the uncovering of meaningful insights. Ethics and participant protection were made a priority while coding and data analysis contributed to the rigour and validity of the study. These elements form a robust and comprehensive research project that captures the perspectives of survivors and the MHPs who support them.

Chapter Five

Results From Study One: Adult Survivors of SPA

The extended literature review performed for these studies (Refer to Chapter Three) reported a dearth of information regarding treatment protocols administered by MHPs to survivors. In addition, the extended literature review reported a scarcity of information regarding the perspectives of survivors receiving treatment from MHPs for SPA abuse.

Chapter Five, 'Results From Study One', comprises survivor demographics, social dimensions and CITs reported by survivors, frequent topics arising from the study interviews, and the six key emerging themes within these concurrent studies. The choice to research the perspectives of survivors who work with MHPs (Volume Two) was exploratory and sought to obtain new data on this topic to expand on the limited existing and comparable research. Currently, most data pertain to children of PA, not adult survivors of PA, SPA or SPAA.

At the conclusion of Chapter Five, Volume Two, the subsequent chapter, Chapter Six, titled 'Results From Study Two: Mental Health Practitioners,' will present an examination of the perspectives provided by MHPs specialising in working therapeutically with survivors. Following Chapter Six, Chapter Seven will introduce the discussion and conclusion from Study One, focusing on survivors' perspectives of working with MHPs.

Additionally, Chapter Eight will report on the discussion and conclusion of Study Two regarding the perspectives of MHPs who work with survivors. These distinct chapters, Chapter Seven and Chapter Eight, will analyse and discuss the outcomes of both studies in detail. Both 'Discussion and Conclusion' sections will integrate the insights from both studies, offering a comprehensive overview of the research findings. Future research suggestions and contributions to these studies are also presented.

Adult Survivor Study Participants

Table One, titled 'Adult Survivor Participant Demographics' on the following page, includes the participants' country of origin, gender, age at their parents' separation or divorce, their TPs gender, and the length of separation from the TP. Additionally, the table details whether the adult survivor was moved away as a child, was withheld, or abducted by their AP interstate or internationally, away from their TP. Furthermore, the table includes data on whether the survivors have alienated children themselves.

TABLE TWO

Adult Survivor Participant Demographics

Participants identifying letter, Age and Country where they live	Sex	Age at parents' divorce or separation	Sex of the targeted parent	Length of separation from the targeted parent	Has/had alienated children themselves	Was moved away, withheld, abducted interstate or abducted internationally from the targeted parent
K 32 America	F	8	Father	10 years	Yes-current	Withheld
A 53 America	F	2	Father	44 years	No	Yes-interstate
A 54 Australia	M	7	Father	12 years, then no contact for another 14 years, then no contact again.	Yes-Current	Yes-interstate
B 42 Indigenous Australia	F	2	Father	15 years	No	Withheld
M 21 Canada	F	5	Mother	8 years	No	Withheld

M 19 Canada	M	8	Mother	8 years	No	Withheld
A 1- 49 Australia	M	10	Mother	No data	Yes-previously	International
A 61 America	F	10	Mother	15 years	No	No data
T 46 United Kingdom	M	2	Father	28	Yes-current	Withheld
S 55 Germany	M	8	Father	10	No	Withheld
J 45 Australia	F	11	Father	10	Yes	Taken away

The following sub-theme reports on data results obtained from the twenty-one interviews. The twenty-one interviews comprised eleven survivors in the first cohort (n=11) and ten MHPs (n=10) in the second cohort. Of these eleven participants, seven identified as women, and four identified as men. One of the adult participants was interviewed for the two concurrent studies as they met the criteria by identifying as an adult survivor of SPA and a clinical psychologist.

Including a participant who met the criteria of being both an adult survivor of SPA and a clinical psychologist for the two concurrent studies introduced a potential bias in the data. This participant's dual role provided a unique perspective, combining personal experience as a survivor with professional expertise as an MHP, which has not been recorded before. As a result, their responses and insights might have influenced the findings and interpretations of the studies.

To address this potential bias, the Researcher took several precautions during the research process. Firstly, the participant's data was treated with the same rigour and objectivity as other participants. Their responses were analysed alongside those of other participants to identify common themes and patterns. Secondly, the Researcher implemented stringent research methodologies, ensuring that data collection and analysis procedures remained consistent across all participants. This helped minimise the potential influence of the participant's dual role on the findings.

The research report disclosed the participant's unique status as a survivor and an MHP to provide transparency. However, this information was not disclosed to the researchers who conducted the blind interview analysis to enable an unbiased evaluation of the data. By acknowledging and addressing this potential bias, the Researcher aimed to maintain the integrity and validity of the study's findings. The Researcher collated and analysed the data separately under two studies and two study cohorts. For more information regarding the MHPs cohort interview results, please refer to Chapter Six.

Social Dimensions and Complex Intersecting Traumas

Previous research examined the existing literature on trauma and explored CITs encountered by survivors who have experienced "other similar types of abuse." Chapter Two of the study discusses these CITs under "Related Parallel Trauma." It is crucial for MHPs working with survivors to be aware of CITs. Since there is limited research on survivors in this area, the study draws upon 'similar types of abuse' to fill this research gap. Some areas considered for these studies include childhood sexual abuse, child abduction, abandonment, dissociation and abuse, Stockholm syndrome, and familicide. Stockholm syndrome is mentioned because the child's profound attachment to the alienating mother (in this case) is occasionally likened to Stockholm syndrome, wherein the child develops an emotional or symbiotic bond to cope with the psychological pressure exerted by the AP (Montagna, 2019). For example, to restore their sense of worthiness in the eyes of the AP, the alienated child may adopt the behaviours and attitudes of the AP (Fares et al., 2023). Consequently, it becomes crucial for the child to maintain a negative emotional climate when in the presence of the AP, as this fosters trust and approval from the AP (Fares et al., 2023).

Additionally, these studies present data collected explicitly on CITs experienced by the study participants, eliminating the need to rely on related parallel trauma areas as was done during the extended literature review. In addition, this collection of CITs will add to the dearth of literature available on survivors for MHPs to draw upon therapeutically.

Previous research suggests that survivors may seek therapy with a 'disguised presentation' instead of for treatment about their child abuse encounter per se (Gelinas, 1983). Gelinas's (1983) research results were replicated in the data gathered from participants in these studies. For example, survivors stated that they only learned about SPA later in life even though they had been seeking help from MHPs for underlying and confusing symptoms for many years. Survivors also reported that MHPs they had sought help from did not notice or mention that their symptoms were linked to child abuse and SPA. Based on the declarations made by numerous survivors in these studies regarding their experiences with CITs, it is reasonable to assume that the same holds for survivors who sought support from other MHPs to address symptoms related to SPA.

Consequently, these results encouraged the Researcher to investigate the MHP data (cohort two) to cross-compare answers regarding their perspectives on survivor symptomology and disguised presentations (Gelinas, 1983) survivors during a session. For example, "MHP1" explained that "many of their colleague practitioners focused solely on treating the symptoms experienced by survivors rather than addressing the underlying SPA itself". Furthermore, "MHP1" noted that "adult survivors can often present with an array of concerning physical symptoms".

Results

Frequent Topics Arising from Interviews with Adult Survivors

Six main themes were identified under the primary theme of 'Survivor perspectives on therapies applied by a mental health practitioner for treatment of SPA'. These six themes were chosen because they were the highest-ranked 'frequent topic' in the following thematic discussion listed in Figure Three.

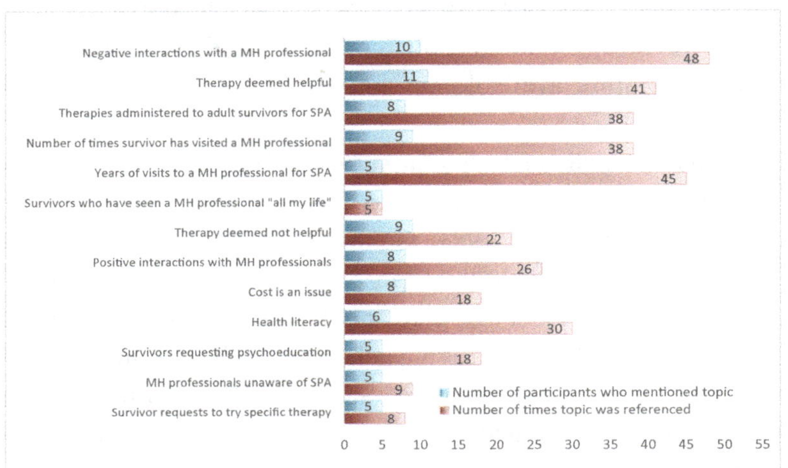

FIGURE THREE

'Frequent Topics' Arising from Data Collected from Adult Survivors of SPA

Note: Figure Three shows the 'frequent topics' (in graduated blue) revealed by survivors during their interviews. The graduated tan line represents the number of times the survivors referenced the 'frequent topic' during the interviews. The topics were ranked in importance from highest to lowest, starting with the most significant digit difference between the frequent topics and the number of times the frequent topics were expressed during interviews.

Thematic Discussion

Key Emerging Themes

This chapter summarises the six key emerging data themes and describes examples of adult survivor experiences and perspectives gathered during the research interviews. Survivor participants have been deidentified to protect their confidentiality. The six key themes that have emerged from the data collected from survivors are listed in Figure Four.

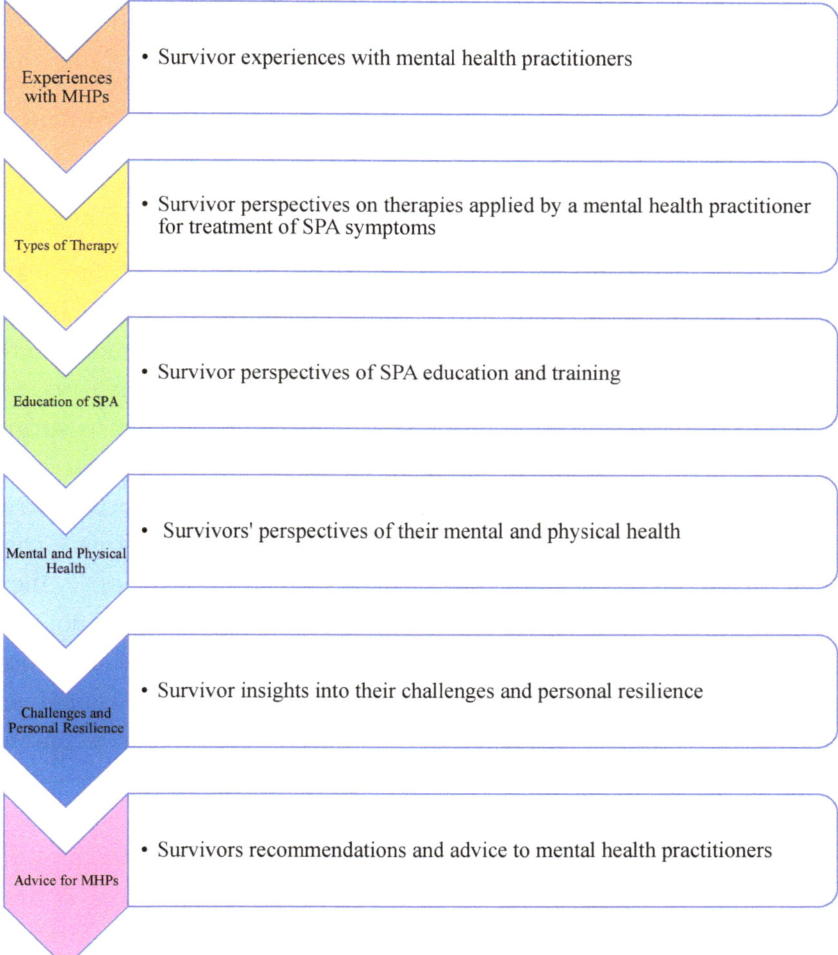

Experiences with MHPs
• Survivor experiences with mental health practitioners
Types of Therapy
• Survivor perspectives on therapies applied by a mental health practitioner for treatment of SPA symptoms
Education of SPA
• Survivor perspectives of SPA education and training
Mental and Physical Health
• Survivors' perspectives of their mental and physical health
Challenges and Personal Resilience
• Survivor insights into their challenges and personal resilience
Advice for MHPs
• Survivors recommendations and advice to mental health practitioners

FIGURE FOUR

Main Themes Emerging from Adult Survivor Data

Study Prerequisites

The Researcher requested that interested participants complete the Baker Strategy Questionnaire (BSQ) (Baker & Chambers, 2011) for inclusion in the study. Participants who mainly scored 4's (4 representing the most severe experiences of SPA as opposed to 1, 2 or 3 being lesser traumatic experience scores) participated in the study. The BSQ questions are available to view in Appendix Five.

Data Analysis

All interviews were conducted via the secure USC Zoom platform. Interview data were transcribed verbatim and entered into a Word document uploaded into NVivo 12. Participants' data were de-identified for the reporting objectives using an iterative review process (Horsfall & Pinn, 2009). Key factors contributing to survivors' perspectives were identified from the data gathered and categorised by the Researcher and three fellow academic researchers. Two researchers were from The University of the Sunshine Coast (USC) (DR and WK), and the third researcher was from Sydney University (KCG). These three reviewers, all of whom are doctors and researchers, conducted a comprehensive examination and meticulous review of the transcribed text. After conversations and an agreed consensus, subsequent transcripts were submitted to a content analysis in which each distinctive group of thoughts were separated from the original transcript and coded. For example, how long have you been attending sessions for SPA with MHPs? What therapies do you remember undertaking? Were they helpful? If not, why? A first and second round pass of qualitative data coding was performed, then organised into qualitative codes and subcodes. Further rounds of coding were performed until key themes and sub-themes emerged from the repeated words and phrases.

Participants' Employment and Education

Ten of the eleven participants were employed at the time of the interview.

Bachelor's Degree

Within the adult survivor cohort, three participants were studying for a bachelor's degree in psychology. Additionally, one survivor was studying a double major in women's and gender studies and sociology, which included conducting research interviews. Interestingly, six participants hold ten bachelor's degrees between them. These degrees are nursing, art history criticism and conversation, horticulture, criminal justice and victimology, computer science and information systems, cyber security, law, music, physiotherapy, and psychology.

Master's Degree

Also, within the adult survivor cohort, four participants have six master's degrees between them. These degrees are clinical psychology, teaching-secondary English- modern history and visual art methods, education, special education and teaching, criminal justice management, and business administration.

Doctoral Degree

In addition, one study participant holds a doctorate in clinical psychology.

Results of Survivors' Degrees

The combined degrees total seventeen completed degrees among six survivors and three pending degrees for the three bachelor-level student participants. Once the pending undergraduate degrees are complete, the total will add up to nine participants out of eleven who have completed a university degree. Interestingly, once the current three bachelor-level student participants have graduated, the total number of degrees will add up to twenty between eleven participants. The following Key Theme One discusses the main themes emerging from adult survivor data regarding their perspectives and experiences with MHPs.

KEY THEME ONE

Survivor Experiences with MHPs

Survivors who participated in the study were keen to discuss their perspectives and experiences regarding time spent seeking support for challenges and CITs associated with SPA with MHPs and health professionals. Please note that the term 'professionals' within these studies refers to people who work in mental health but are not qualified practitioners. For example, 'professionals' equals- youth workers, social workers, mental health nurses, peer workers, occupational therapists, doctors/general practitioners, psychiatrists, developmental psychologists, and forensic psychologists. 'MHPs' in the context of these studies are accredited MH professionals with a degree in clinical psychotherapy, general and clinical psychology, and psychiatry with a master's degree in counselling. Some of the study participants have seen various MH professionals, and when this is the case, the applicable term is applied for clarification.

Negative Experiences with MHPs

Within this sub-theme, negative experiences with MHPs were a key theme emerging from the interviews. All participants had a strong sense of not feeling understood, being judged, worrying about the practitioners' reaction to their trauma stories and feeling they may be abandoned if they became 'too hard to work with' during a session.

All eleven participants identified that they had experienced negative encounters with MHPs, with forty-eight references to negative experiences being coded and analysed for inclusion. All participants displayed a high level of awareness regarding the impact of SPA on their lives, discussing links between finding out that they were survivors of SPA and when they started on their healing journey. Also, participants discussed links between finding an MHP whose reaction they do not have to worry about and the possibility of having to regulate the therapists themselves during a session.

Furthermore, having to figuratively wear their own mask in therapy to protect themselves from the therapist not believing them was also communicated. Survivors explained the challenges they faced from practitioners when they shared their stories of trauma. For example, according to the practitioner, the following participant experienced surprise when she told her MHP that her story of trauma and how she explained it was not in the normal range. This participant was also shocked that the therapist had such a visceral reaction to her story;

> I've seen one lady two times. And she says, oh, can you give me a little bit of a background so I kind of know where you've come from? And then I told her that Mum had died, and I just continued talking. She's just like, whoa, whoa, hang on a minute! You've just said something that is so tragic, but you've just continued on. And that was what woke me up. Here, I am talking about something that's totally rattled her. And she said, look, I'm struggling here. Sometimes, you've got to understand the impact that it has on other people that what you've experienced isn't normal. To me, it was normal, though. (Interviewee Antje-Renee)

This participant's account described a space of surprise and understanding that her reactions were not in the normal range. The inability of MHPs to cope with trauma stories from survivors was evident in this example. Survivors in these studies explained that regulating practitioners enabled them not to be re-victimised if the practitioner was not skilled enough to notice what was happening to the adult survivor. Other survivors were tired of regulating people and strongly voiced their opinions;

> The hardest part for my therapist was being in shock when they got another piece of my story. Because I'm a child of SPA and was abducted, so each time, they were like, WOW, are you kidding? I didn't see my father for 44 years. I've been in grief my whole life. I hated their reaction. I felt victimised all over again. I watch them closely, and they need to wrap their heads around this because I'm sick of regulating people. We're gonna throw a tonne of shit at them, sorry, so they better be ready to do their job. (Interviewee Aurora)

Previous research reports that it does not matter how experienced an MHP is. Hearing recounts of trauma may evoke strong reactions and feelings (Herman, 1992). However, an MHP's capacity to not counter-transfer is based on personal and professional considerations (Wilson & Thomas, 2004). Personal factors for practitioners include their experience in containment, temperament, and resistance to sensitivity and stress. Professional factors include the practitioners' levels of experience and knowledge of trauma, access and availability of resources and support and one's own psychological state (Wilson & Thomas, 2004).

Psychological Safety with MHPs

Survivors' not feeling psychologically safe in sessions with practitioners was reported as problematic. Survivors also described the concern that the practitioner might lack professional knowledge of SPA and struggle to build trust while keeping them safe enough to tell the truth during a session. One survivor shared their experience, stating;

> The first time I saw a therapist, I didn't really open up. I don't think she understood me. And we went on and on. And I began

> to wear a mask. She had a specific type of view or manner that she was trying to maybe push on me. She felt that I was going in the direction that I should start working on myself so that I could work out how to help my mother more. She didn't want to hear the real story, even though my alienating mother was very abusive. So, she kept on persisting. The therapist brought certain biases or prejudices with her (Interviewee Shane) (The Researcher employed a professional German translator in Australia for this interview).

Interestingly, this participants' intuitive comment regarding the therapist bringing in their own biases was validated previously in research explaining that practitioners' reactions are based on personal beliefs and characteristics stemming from sociocultural myths, standards, and personal expectations (Alaggia, 2010; Sorsoli et al., 2008). The same participant also shared that professional therapeutic help when they were a child was not forthcoming as the survivor suspected the practitioner of colluding with his mother and felt that they were not open to listening to his side of the story. He now believes that his general lack of trust, his ongoing hearing problems and the dissociation he experiences have all contributed to the suicidality he lives with as an adult male, as shared through the following extract;

> My mother was abusive, and the therapist believed her and what my mother was telling the therapist about my father. The therapist asked me, "And what's about the stories about your father? I think they're all true." For ten years as a child, every day, hearing bad things about my father being bad. I was told you are bad like your father, and your father does these terrible things to you. I was told that my father sexually abused me when he didn't. For years, my mother screamed at me in my room at night that my father had sex with me. The therapist didn't hear me. She only listened to what Mum said.

> Now I get hearing problems, and then I got dissociation. I lost trust in her because you cannot be as suicidal as I am and hear anymore that you are guilty. It's too dangerous for me. (Interviewee Shane) (The Researcher employed a professional German translator in Australia for this session).

Clients Teaching Insider Knowledge of SPA

Within this sub-theme, survivors reported feeling abandoned and worried that their new practitioner might also leave. Participants in these studies described that she had taught practitioners about SPA to stop being abandoned. "Aurora" explained that she taught the practitioner insider knowledge of SPA (knowledge that only a survivor would have on their trauma) and hoped that these teachings would get the MHP to pay more attention to their stories, which may stop them from leaving. "Aurora" also described that the downside made her feel like a guinea pig. Aurora also explained that she was getting nothing out of treatment and paying to get the help that was never coming, and the practitioner learnt a lot about PA and SPA at their expense. "Aurora" had also shared that she continued this pattern for a long time and that "it was better help than no help at all. Previous research reports that disclosures of abuse that are met negatively by MHPs can result in secondary victimisation (Ahrens et al., 2010). Secondary victimisation can last long after the abuse has finished (Ahrens et al., 2010). The following is an example from another study participant who shared her perspectives on feeling abandoned by their therapist;

> It felt a bit like I was being abandoned when my last therapist left. The excuse they gave me was that therapists are just leaving in droves at the moment; they're burnt out. With my new therapist, it's clear that she's pregnant, so sooner or later, we're going to have to have that conversation about what we're going to do there. But that's a battle I don't need to fight today. I feel it's exhausting retelling my story." (Interviewee Jane)

Another survivor described how she has had to develop skills to explain her personal story of SPA to lay people around her so that they understood her trauma. She also shared her experience working with her current MHPs and the lengths she has had to go to reach a point where she feels understood in the following extract;

> Because, for so many friends and people around me, I've had to explain this experience and make it make sense for others, which, I mean, is a real task. I do feel like I have to come in with an explanation prepared and all this background information to explain what the heck it is I'm talking about. You know, I feel like it was pointless. Just make a PowerPoint presentation or something." (Interviewee Marie)

Lost All Hope of Finding Help

Some participants reported a deterioration of hope because they believed they would never recover from their SPA abuse. The participants cited an absence of hope due to a lack of education about SPA for MHPs and feeling they would never find anyone who understands their child abuse trauma. This data indicated a need for self-agency skills to be taught by MHPs to survivors. Self-agency education refers to the "development of internal representations of being an active, effective agent in the world, including the interpersonal world" (Brown & Elliot, 2016, p. 627). Experiences accompanying self-agency development variations regarding mastery and self-efficacy are described as helplessness, hopelessness, and ineffectiveness (Brown & Elliot, 2016, p. 626). Any participants within this sub-theme did not report self-agency skills. Adverse experiences shared by participants were linked to a lack of hope that they would find an MHP they could trust and understand them. For example, the following extract from the perspective of "Shane", who describes how practitioners they have received treatment from seemed to have no understanding, training or knowledge regarding SPA, which left them feeling traumatised and abandoned;

> I feel like the only person that can really help me is myself, unfortunately. The ones that I was able to see and participate in and have sessions with is that none of them were beneficial to me. It was almost as if they were trying to change my mind about how I felt and make me think something that wasn't the truth. And I know it wasn't the truth. It was as if they were trying to paint a different picture and rewrite my childhood or what I physically remember, what I'd physically seen, and make me feel a way that wasn't how I was feeling. Sadly, I can't say that any of them helped me at all. (Interviewee Shane) (The Researcher employed a professional German translator in Australia for this interview).

In the following extract, "Marie" elaborated on the theme of 'lost all hope' by explaining how she does not think SPA can ever be stopped and how it will stay with her for her entire life;

> I don't know if there's anything that can ever be done to stop it. I don't know if there's enough education out there that psychologists and therapists and trauma therapists can do. It's a lifelong thing, and it sticks with you. And it influences your entire being because a lot of this experience is when we're really young. And so that impacts us while we're still developing. So, of course, it's going to be around for our entire lives. I think it can have very long-lasting effects on life. (Interviewee Marie)

In the following extract, "Antje-Renee" described the traumatic encounter she had experienced in the practitioner's office. "You're kind of going in this one-hour appointment. I don't want to walk out of there feeling like I've been emotionally raped. Because yes, that's what I felt like when I had that appointment with that psychologist". Another participant named "Alan" also shared how practitioners have not helped him during therapeutic sessions. "I'd say the one-on-one classic psychotherapist-patient relationship hour sessions/ 50-minute sessions, whatever the case may be, maybe one has helped out of many."

Aurora's Poignant Reflection

In the following extract, "Aurora", a study participant and adult survivor of SPAA, offers readers a unique glimpse into her personal experiences and perspective regarding therapeutic support for her childhood trauma. These study participants provide valuable insights into the complex realities faced by individuals who access MHPs for help, shedding light on the profound impact it has had on their life;

> Therapists who understand us are nowhere to be found, and even when we think that we can trust someone, I find that I am too much for them. After a while of nodding, taking my money and not much help, they looked overwhelmed and confused and ended our sessions. This left me feeling abandoned, rejected, crazy, unable to be helped and a lost cause. (Aurora)

This poignant reflection resonates with a more extensive concern identified within the literature. As "Aurora" expresses her struggles to find MHPs who comprehend the complexities of her trauma, her sentiments highlight a prevailing issue faced by many survivors. The following topic reports on survivor perspectives of therapies that MHPs have applied to help with their trauma.

KEY THEME TWO

Survivor Perspectives on Therapies Applied by an MHP for the Treatment of SPA

Survivors' perspectives on therapeutic SPA treatments were linked to many trial-and-error therapy experiences. For example, across the eleven survivors interviewed, eight reported forty-one different references to the question, "What types of therapy was tried or suggested by the practitioner to help you with your SPA symptoms?" Please refer to the following Table Three for a comprehensive list of therapies provided to survivors.

TABLE THREE

Therapies Applied by MHPs to Adult Survivors as Stated by Adult Survivors

Therapies Applied
Generalised counselling
Massage therapy
Grief therapy
Reunification therapy with the TP
Tapping
Family therapy
Collating art and craft images
Journalling
Neuro linguistic programming
Timestamp therapy
Inner child therapy
Cognitive behaviour therapy
Mirror work therapy
Self-talk therapy
Self-love therapy
Attachment styles
Avoidance therapy
People pleasing
Dealing with trauma
Trauma-informed work
Abandonment

Unconditional positive regard
Reframing thoughts
Psychodynamic therapy
Working intrinsically instead of extrinsically
Dealienation programming
Life and relationship coaching
Reiki
Wrapping your body mentally in colours
Compartmentalising
Drawing pictures
Reunification therapy
Brain spotting
Homework with topics to work on and bring back to therapy
Child development
Emotionally focused therapy
Eye movement desensitisation and reprocessing therapy
Art therapy
Nature therapy
Exercise therapy
Group therapy

The list of therapies applied by MHPs to survivors underscores the need for evidence-based treatment models and holistic therapies to guide practitioners in their work. In addition, the fact that survivors reported trying multiple therapies highlights the challenges and complexities of treating SPA and the importance of finding the right combination of treatments that will work for the individual survivor.

The list of therapies includes therapies such as cognitive behaviour therapy, eye movement desensitisation and reprocessing therapy, and more holistic approaches, such as massage therapy, nature therapy, and reiki. This personalised preferred treatment view suggests that a combination of medical and holistic approaches may be most effective in treating SPA. The most effective way to test this hypothesis would be in clinical trials with survivors and MHPs.

However, without evidence-based treatment models to guide practitioners, it can be difficult for MHPs to know which therapies to apply and in what combination. In addition, without a protocol, working with survivors can be a challenging trial-and-error approach that can be time-consuming, costly, and emotionally draining for MHPs and survivors. Therefore, developing evidence-based treatment models for SPA combined with affordable SPA education and clinical supervision is critical to ensure practitioners have a clear and effective roadmap while accessing professional support when treating survivors.

Top Ten Compared Results Between MHPs and Adult Survivors

The therapeutic approaches MHPs utilise in working with survivors are extensive, as Table Three outlines. In contrast, the following 'Table Four' provides an insightful overview of 69 ideas, topics, and psychoeducation that survivors found helpful during their therapy sessions. Among the multitude of therapies mentioned, ten key interventions stood out as particularly beneficial, as identified by the survivors in their own words.

These top ten therapies overlapped between the MHPs and survivors: massage work, trauma-informed treatment, psychoeducation, inner child therapy, boundary work, nature therapy, child psychology, abandonment therapy, deprogramming of brainwashing, and group therapy. The survivors expressed a strong desire for MHPs to possess in-depth knowledge of these various topics and emphasised the importance of delivering interventions safely.

Furthermore, the survivors emphasised the need for MHPs to continually build upon their skills and expand their understanding of these therapeutic topics. The survivors stressed that MHPs should effectively implement these interventions during therapy sessions based on the survivors' specific needs and circumstances. The survivors' perspectives highlight the significance of a shared, comprehensive and tailored approach to therapy. They underscore the importance of MHPs acquiring a broad repertoire of therapeutic techniques and a nuanced understanding of the survivors' unique challenges. By integrating the survivors' preferred therapies and topics into their practice, MHPs can create a safe and supportive environment that facilitates the survivors' healing process.

TABLE FOUR

Ideas, Topics, and Psychoeducation as Recommended by Survivors

Ideas, Topics, and Psychoeducation
Domestic violence support
Having clear goals
Help with brainwashing and gaslighting from the AP
Reframing of stories
Boundary setting with alienating parents
Conflict and anxiety around being near the AP
Inner child work
Phobias regarding bringing up topics, especially about the TP around the AP
Learning to say no
Unconditional positive regard
Self-awareness
Identifying triggers and how to move through them safely
Processing of feelings
Stop overthinking and over-reacting
Coping with guilt about parents fighting

Ideas, Topics, and Psychoeducation
Coping with guilt about the way the TP has been treated
Coping with guilt about not regulating the AP
Doing karate
Doing sports in a forest
Learning why certain behaviours exist in survivors
Watching psychoeducation videos on PA
Learning how cults operate to gain an understanding of the AP and how they think
Dealing with step-parents and step-children who may have alienating traits
Reversing brainwashing
Working holistically
Art therapy
Meditation
Painting
Creating images of how they feel in the moment
Learning to speak about emotions
Counteracting feeling dissociated
Music therapy
Learning about emotional detachment disorder
Drama therapy
Learning mediation skills
Yoga Nidra
Learning strategies to compartmentalise
Trauma recovery
Compassion and empathy

Ideas, Topics, and Psychoeducation
Building Immunity to trauma
Finding a therapist who is a confidante
Finding a psychotherapist, not a psychologist
Journaling
Writing on scraps of paper and burning the pieces
Finding special items from childhood and playing with them
Alternatives to violence
Issues with relationships like marriage or kids or career
Massage
Attachment theory training
Abandonment work
Unconditional positive regard
Psychodynamic psychotherapy
Reiki
Reunification therapy
Child psychology
Eye Movement Desensitisation and Reprocessing Therapy
Nature therapy
Exercise therapy
Group therapy
Phobias and paranoia about being harmed
Phobias and paranoia about family members being harmed
Dealing with violence from step-parents and/or their children
Talking about the suicide of a parent or sibling
Talking safely about homicidal ideation regarding the alienating parent/step-parent

Ideas, Topics, and Psychoeducation
Talking safely about revenge against alienating or step-parent
Therapy about difficult medical symptoms
Therapy for physical and/or sexual abuse as children
Psychoeducation about the Family Court System
Therapy for not repeating the child abuse

KEY THEME THREE

Survivor Perspectives of SPA Education and Training for MHPs and Themselves

Within Theme Three, survivor perspectives of SPA education and training for MHPs and themselves were reported. For example, one survivor spoke candidly about feeling confused about why therapists do not understand survivors of SPA and the social dimensions they may have faced when there are millions of survivors of high-conflict divorce worldwide. An example of the consequent level of additional frustration regarding explaining what SPA is to new therapists is described in the following extract;

> I do feel like I have to come in with an explanation prepared and all this background information to explain what the heck it is I'm talking about with a new therapist. So yeah, I definitely do have to put in that effort. I think. It's just a matter of understanding how deep the brainwashing really goes. And how that has an impact on you, like, the cognitive dissonance that that creates. A lot of the time, people I've spoken to don't necessarily understand why my brother and I had felt that way growing up. We had this deep hatred for our mother. (Interviewee Marie)

The table in the following 'Figure Five' displays the data collected from survivors' perspectives regarding the education and training of MHPs who have had therapeutic sessions within the context of SPA. Notably, four of the eleven survivor participants reported the need to educate their MHPs about PA and SPA, as the survivor perceived these professionals as having limited knowledge. Additionally, the survivors reported that they had sought therapy from (approximately) 50 MHPs over the years for help with PA and SPA. However, the survivors perceived that only three were trained in SPA. The figure of approximately 50 was extracted from the interview data and was based on survivors stating an approximate number when asked how many MHPs they had accessed help from over the years.

The graph also highlights the issue of health literacy, with six survivors mentioning this topic 30 times. This data indicates that, on average, the survivors perceived that they possessed a significantly more comprehensive understanding of SPA than most MHPs they interacted with, yet they still had to pay for numerous unhelpful sessions.

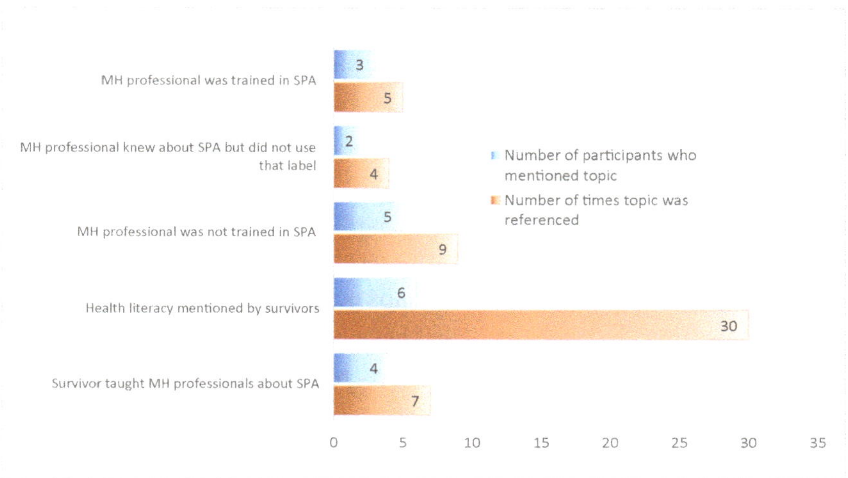

FIGURE FIVE

Survivor Perspectives of SPA Education and Training for MHPs

Despite the limited number of MHPs reported as being helpful, these studies describe that therapy costs remain significant. These studies' data indicate that only three of the numerous MHPs reported by survivors had received training in SPA, yet they were still being charged. This discrepancy raises concerns about the financial burden on survivors seeking specialised therapy for SPA.

Cost of Therapy

This issue of therapy costs is further highlighted by the experience shared by a 42-year-old Indigenous Australian participant. She discusses the 'lifelong' duration of her engagement with MHPs for therapy and the ongoing expenses throughout her journey. This personal account sheds light on the additional challenges marginalised communities face, where the cost of therapy for SPA can be a substantial barrier to accessing much-needed support.;

> I've been accessing therapy in a multitude of ways, particularly in the late '90s and early 2000s. I've got a holistic psychotherapist now. You could argue that I've been in counselling my whole life intermittently, like more on than off. So, I'll say that 22 to 24 years. I would definitely say 18 years of that would be accessing some form of therapy or counselling to be able to maintain and navigate relationships. Costs are a double-edged sword. If I was from a lower socioeconomic area and didn't have a good paying job, I guess I could perhaps access free or subsidised counselling, but because I do have a good paying job and I am educated, I don't have access to a $70 pointless visit. I'm talking about upwards of between $200 and $300 a visit, and over covid, I paid $5,000 to do life and relationship coaching. (Interviewee Brianna)

Therapy and the Australian Medicare System

Within this sub-theme, one study participant shared their insights about accessing the Australian Medicare System for counselling. This participant gave his perspectives regarding the limitations of therapies offered under Medicare and the constraints he witnessed placed on the MHPs he has accessed for therapy;

> I think people like me are hard, complex, I've got lots of different voices that need speaking to or parts of us that need speaking to or lots of doors that need to be aired, and a light shone into, and I think it's just down to the human on the other side of the room, their capabilities and their experience, I guess, or their gifts, their skill, or what they're limited to providing because I've seen a few of the therapists under a mental health care plan, and they're very limited with the types of therapies that they can employ in those sessions. It's usually just CBT, and I need a lot more than that. (Interviewee Alan)

KEY THEME FOUR (MENTAL HEALTH)

Survivors' Perspectives of Their Mental Health

Mental Health-Identity and Suicidality

Generally, in epidemiological research, the term 'relative risk' relates to the risk of association between the strength of the exposure to disease and the consequence of disease (Flaskerud & Winslow, 2010). In this instance, 'relative risk' applies to the vulnerable population of survivors with an increased risk of illness due to a decreased health status in this research data. None of the adult survivor participants interviewed for this research claimed to have power, money, or access to good healthcare. Unfortunately, Flaskerud and Winslow (2010, p. 298) report that "people without resources are exposed to more and greater risks and, as a consequence, experience worse health status or health disparities." Ideally, the more mental health is discussed regarding treatment resources, the better the health status may be, which may also lead to a decrease in comorbidities within vulnerable people such as the survivors in these studies.

The unwillingness of people within the general community to discuss mental illness is evident in previous research articles, reporting on the predilection to speak to professionals regarding practical tasks such as requesting financial advice instead of discussing mental health (Judd et al., 2006). Despite programs and advertising aimed at encouraging more people to talk about mental health, there is still a stigma attached to a diagnosis of mental illness or when a person displays an inability to cope in their lives. This sub-theme focuses on the mental health difficulties reported by survivors in the study. In the subsequent pages, these

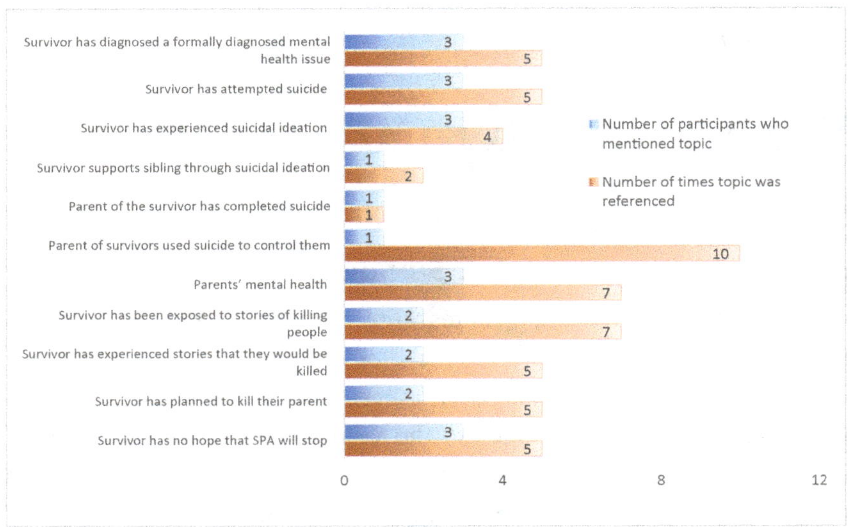

FIGURE SIX

Adult Survivors' Perspectives of their own Mental and Physical Health

survivors clearly describe the impact of these challenges on their physical well-being and daily lives.

Additionally, it is worth noting that 30% of the participants openly shared their formally diagnosed mental health conditions and expressed their thoughts on suicide. Furthermore, the subsequent page delves into the sensitive topics of parental murder and the painful subject of parents who have died by suicide. Finally, the following graph reports on study data gathered from the Survivors' Perspectives on their Mental and Physical Health.

Different Sides of Suicide

The findings of these studies revealed that 50% of the survivors identified that they had thought about and planned to die by suicide. However, they stopped before completion. Furthermore, 30% of the survivors mentioned that they have thought about suicide but would not act on the impulse, and two participants feel that they often have to support their siblings to prevent them from dying by suicide due to SPA.

Regarding the parents of survivors and suicide, one survivor has experienced the tragic suicide of their mother because of SPA, and another survivor's mother used the threat of suicide on many occasions to stop him from contacting his father. This particular mother's threats of suicide were openly displayed in front of the survivor, and he shared the following emotional account;

> It was Christmas day, and I wanted to call my father. I was about 12 or 13. If you do that, said my mother, I'll do something terrible to myself. I said OK, but I really want to call him. After that, she began to burn her house sweater. She took her cigarette lighter and began lighting up her clothes, burning her clothes that she was wearing. I try to stop her, but she had set herself alight. I had to pour water over her to put her out. (Interviewee Shane) (The Researcher

> employed a professional German translator in Australia for this interview).

The participant's life took a significant turn due to this event, as the threat prevented him from ever asking to speak to his father.

False Allegations of Child Sexual Abuse

The participant explained that because of the false allegations of sexual abuse that his mother had been accusing his father of doing to him for so long, he didn't trust his father, even though he couldn't ever remember it happening. However, this did not stop him from wanting to push past his feelings of low self-esteem due to his internal drive to call his father. Previous research explains that this was a tough barrier for this participant to push through because adults who lack a well-developed sense of self-agency usually feel ineffective and powerless (Brown & Elliot, 2016). In addition, these adults tend to be passive-dependent, allowing others to decide what they need and how to get it (Brown & Elliot, 2016).

This participant then shared the following attempt to contact his father after waiting a couple of years and when he finally felt safe enough to re-express his desire to call his father at age 16. This survivor managed to intuitively draw strength from within himself and then pose the request to speak to his father again to his mother, hoping to gain a different response this time. Unfortunately, the mother rejected this request, and he was again exposed to SPA and family violence as his punishment. This request refusal reversed his self-agency to passive dependence (Brown & Elliot, 2016). This time, the mother instantly began the same pattern regarding threats of suicide. However, she escalated her behaviour and actively chose to run from the house and scare him at a greater level than just setting herself on fire;

> I was a shadow. I wasn't brave, but I wanted to go beyond my feelings. Then I think it was also Christmas. I don't forget

> the burning, but I want to call my father. I have to. And she started to tell me something about suicide and what she would do if I were to call my father. She was just in her underwear in the kitchen. Suddenly, she runs out into the snowy weather. She runs straight toward the train station. She wants to jump before the train! But I catch her 10 metres before the train. She was lying there. I told her she was safe. Then she started laughing like crazy at me and laughed, you poor bad boy. It was like etched into me or burnt into me. So, I didn't dare to do anything after that. Whether she would actually have done it or not. I don't know whether it was true. (Interviewee Shane) (The Researcher employed a professional German translator in Australia for this interview).

False allegations of CSA can have significant and long-lasting effects on survivors, particularly when these allegations come from a trusted caregiver or family member (Cashmore & Shackel, 2013). Survivors may feel various emotions, including stigmatisation, social isolation, and vulnerability (Finkelhor & Browne, 1985). These false allegations can also profoundly impact their self-esteem and sense of identity, leading to a feeling of powerlessness and loss of agency (Finkelhor & Browne, 1985).

Survivors may also experience difficulty forming healthy relationships due to these false allegations and may struggle with trusting others or feel as though they are constantly under suspicion or scrutiny (Finkelhor & Browne, 1985). These feelings can be compounded by the lack of understanding or support from others, such as friends, family members, or mental health professionals (Finkelhor & Browne, 1985).

In some cases, false allegations of CSA can also result in legal or criminal proceedings, which can have further negative consequences for the survivor. They may experience additional trauma and stress associated with the legal process and feelings of guilt, shame, and stigma associated with being accused of a crime (Finkelhor & Browne, 1985). Furthermore, false allegations of CSA can impact survivors' and their families' mental health and well-being by straining relationships, leading to a breakdown in communication, trust, and support (Finkelhor & Browne, 1985).

It is important to recognise the significant impact that false allegations of CSA can have on survivors and to provide them with the support and resources they need to address the trauma associated with these experiences. Treatment may involve trauma-informed counselling, advocacy, legal support, and educating the broader community about the impact of false allegations on survivors and their families. By providing effective support and resources to survivors, we can help to promote healing, resilience, and recovery.

Many of the participants in the study commented on their 'perspectives of their own mental and physical health' and how important it was that they kept working toward healing solutions. "Alan" shared about his struggle with suicidality in his late teens and how he tries to manage these thoughts now. "Alan" also shared that he does not hate his life anymore because he has put a value on himself by giving himself a new 'identity' to help his own healing from the ingrained trauma patterns;

> Suicidality played a big role when I was younger, and I still feel its pull, but I see it for what it is now. But yes, I've had a rifle nozzle in my mouth, gun loaded, and safety off, but just didn't follow through on the final piece of that puzzle, and that was when I was about 19, 20. Just self-loathing, really, that was the core of it. So, I don't hate me anymore. I'm still trying to heal in my 50's. Now I'm doing gardening. I've lived in this house for over two decades, 25 years, and I never gave a rat's arse about my garden. I've put value in myself and my surroundings, my environment, to actually make some changes to it that I want to do, rather than have one foot out

> the door ready to flee because that's how I was brought up. That's what I learned. I did everything I was told. I had no identity. (Interviewee Alan)

Within these studies, 40% of participants reported having a diagnosed mental health condition. The percentages divided into acquainted to 10% mentioned dissociation and anxiety. Another referenced ADHD and emotional attachment disorder. The third reported anxiety and depression, CPTSD and nervous system dysregulation, and the fourth participant spoke about their lifelong struggle with anxiety, depression and CPTSD. Others in the study reported that they had discussions with professionals regarding a never-formalised diagnosis.

Identity and Suicidality

Two participants spoke about the role of identity being linked to what was required of them from their AP. These participants commented on the need to appease the parent, leaving them feeling unsafe, suicidal and with no identity. The need for identity being linked to suicidality was a connection that featured two men and one woman in the study. One participant explained how difficult the paradox they found themselves living in was when they tried to die by suicide. They shared that all of the years of his AP came into his room, ripping off the bed sheets and accusing his TP of sexually abusing him after a contact visit had never been true and had never left him. The survivor discovered the truth after the AP was on their deathbed and told the survivor they had made it up, and his TP was actually a nice guy. After years of terrifying stories, ending his life was the only way out of the "etched pain in his brain" that he still felt as an adult. This story of enmeshment and brainwashing was present in many of the participants in the study, and some participants shared their daily struggles, the cognitive dissonance they felt, and how they needed to live as adults without dying by suicide. The quote below highlights the level of complexity and thought that goes into planning to die by suicide due to lifelong narratives being told to one survivor by his mother;

> I'm sitting in the window of a high building, and I want to die, but I realised that I cannot because I have to still care about my mother. You have to lose the care, and so it's so branded in my mind. Etched. I don't see anything. It all went black. My last thought was that I can't die because I've got to help my mother even though she had done all those things to me, and it was always the same. It was always like that. So, I always defined my own self-esteem by the state or condition of my mother. So, this person that had done all those things to me, I still wanted to help her so I couldn't kill myself. (Interviewee Shane) (The Researcher employed a professional German translator in Australia for this interview).

Another participant revealed the alignment of his mother with the therapist he was being taken to see as a young child;

> I have a good therapist now. And we are working on that suicide point on many points because if you believe that your father has done these things, you will not trust him. My early therapist always aligned with my mother. I had to do what the therapist told me to do, which was looking after my mother. She didn't listen to me. (Interviewee Shane) (The Researcher employed a professional German translator in Australia for this interview).

Finally, the last participant to share about suicide reported haunted, paranoid wonderings about what it would be like to die by suicide and the personal realisations regarding the trauma she had endured;

> On several occasions, I felt like I just wanted to stop existing and what it would be like to just not be here." This was the

> trauma, anxiety and paranoia talking, and this is definitely an area that the right trauma-informed therapy can address. After having kids, I stopped having those thoughts, but I struggle with phobias and paranoia. (Interviewee Aurora)

Aurora's experience with parenting brought a significant shift in her thoughts, but it also led her to grapple with a different challenge- the persistent presence of paranoia.

Phobia and Paranoia Due to Specific Phobia-Anxiety Variant

During the extended literature review, the Researcher discovered a mention of a specific type of phobia called "specific phobia anxiety variant" in an ABPA literature source by Childress (2015). This particular anxiety variant focused on younger children who had experienced the psychological abuse of SPA. However, despite searching for other references in the literature related to PA or SPA, the Researcher could not locate any other sources discussing this specific variant.

With many intriguing questions linking back to the previously mentioned anxiety variant at the forefront of the Researchers' mind, a fascinating discovery emerged among the study participants survivors who had potentially experienced SPAA, FDIOA and SDD as children under the age of eight. These studies' results revealed that survivors impacted by the "specific phobia-severe parental alienation and abduction anxiety variant" (Price-Tobler, 2023) could clearly describe their anxiety and phobia symptoms linked to their SPAA experience as young children under eight. Many survivors informed the Researcher that they still feel many of the phobic, anxious symptoms as adults, and this study was the first time they had spoken about it. Furthermore, the researcher discovered that 75% of the study participants shared experiences and descriptions similar to the researcher's own history of SPAA.

Discovering and identifying this "specific phobia-severe parental alienation and abduction anxiety variant" (Price-Tobler, 2023) positively impacted the Researcher. For example, the resonance between the experiences of the study participants and the Researcher's own lived experience history of SPAA added depth and relevance to her understanding of the topic while validating her previously undocumented (in the academic literature) experience as a child of SPAA.

This personal discovery also filled in a missing puzzle piece for the Researcher that previous MHPs had not noticed during her therapy, and if they did, they had never mentioned it. This resonance added a unique dimension to the Researcher's comprehension of the subject matter, fostering a heightened interest and dedication to further exploring and investigating this new variant. This observation, built from the Researcher's previous investigation into the "specific phobia-anxiety variant" by Childress (2015), constituted a significant discovery and paid homage to the illustrious phrase "Standing on the Shoulders of Invisible Giants" (Elshaikh, n.d).

To support this finding further, the Researcher undertook an extensive search of the peer-reviewed and grey literature on PA, SPA and SPAA to no avail. The Researcher also purchased all available textbooks from Australia and internationally on specific phobias. For example, "Overcoming Specific Phobia, A Hierarchy and Exposure-Based Protocol for the Treatment of all Specific Phobias" (Bourne, 1998) and "Specific Phobias, Clinical Applications of Evidence-Based Psychotherapy" (Bruce & Sanderson, 1998) were purchased. However, none of these sources mentioned the "specific phobia-anxiety variant" (Childress, 2015) that Dr Childress had written about. The Researcher hypothesised that perhaps Dr Childress had discovered the "specific phobia anxiety variant", which is why he had written about this variant in his book "Foundations".

To gain additional insights to support the previous hypothesis and validate the new "specific phobia-severe parental alienation and abduction anxiety variant" data (Price-Tobler, 2023), the Researcher contacted Dr Childress directly. The Researcher also requested this meeting to prevent any research bias by offering to explain the complete transparency of her research methods and processes surrounding the discovery of her new variant to Dr Childress, especially because she was incorporating his "specific phobia-anxiety variant" discovery to build upon her research.

The meeting occurred virtually between the Researcher in Sydney, Australia, and Dr Childress in America at 9 am on Tuesday, June 6th (EST), 2023. Dr Childress was in his clinic at 219 N Indian Hill Blvd #201, Claremont, CA 91711, United States. Once the Researcher explained that her "specific phobia-severe parental alienation, and abduction anxiety variant" research had developed from his "specific phobia-anxiety variant" discovery, Dr Childress explained that "he had developed the specific phobia-anxiety variant for young children experiencing ABPA in his clinic". He further explained that "he developed his variant by analysing the diagnostic indicators in the DSM-5". Dr Childress also clarified "that while numerous phobias are listed in the DSM-5, there is no specific phobia related to fathers or mothers due to the protective nature of the attachment system" (C. Childress, personal communication. June 6th, 2023). "Therefore, if a child exhibits symptoms of paranoia toward a parent, it is essential to consider the possibility of a shared delusional disorder" (C. Childress, personal communication. June 6th, 2023).

Validation of the New Variant

During this conversation, Dr Childress expanded on his clinical observations regarding the "specific phobia-anxiety variant" he wrote about in 2015. After Dr Childress listened to how the Researcher discovered the new variant and how she analysed and coded the data, the Researcher and Dr Childress compared the origin and development of each variant and their identifying links and features. Dr Childress recognised and acknowledged that the "specific phobia-severe parental alienation and abduction anxiety variant" (Price-Tobler, 2023) is a previously unrecognised subcategory and a brand new significant scientific discovery that builds on his previous findings (C. Childress, personal communication. June 6th, 2023).

Furthermore, it is important to note that previous literature, such as Gardner's (2008) work, reported extreme levels of hostility, including paranoid delusions and groundless fears of harm or murder, in children affected by some cases of SPA, which were similar to what the survivors in these studies have described. However, it was unclear from Gardner's' (2008) case studies what age the children were and whether actual abductions had occurred in conjunction with the child's SPA trauma. In contrast, the current study's findings shed light on the experiences of survivors affected by the "specific phobia-severe parental alienation and abduction anxiety variant" (Price-Tobler, 2023). For example, these studies' survivors faced severe threats of personal harm and had been abducted by their AP, marking a significant distinction from the participants in Gardner's previous SPA research.

Contradictions in the Literature

Furthermore, the research revealed an interesting contradiction to the descriptions Warshak (2013) provided in the previous literature on children experiencing SPA. Warshak emphasised extreme hostility, defiance, and disobedience exhibited by children experiencing SPA. However, in the current study, the Researcher discovered that survivors impacted by the "specific phobia-severe parental alienation and abduction anxiety variant" (Price-Tobler, 2023) reported that they would never have confronted their TP in anger or defiance and would shut down and withdraw to protect themselves from further abuse from their AP instead. The survivors were adamant in their responses and stated that they believed the previous research about them being aggressive, hostile, disobedient, and arrogant was incorrect.

Furthermore, the survivors explained that due to experiencing anxious and phobic symptoms due to severe threats of personal harm, including abduction, kidnapping, or being killed, conveyed to them by their AP, they never had their own voice as children and were never taught to stand up for themselves. One survivor "Alan" explained that "saying anything that went against my mother (AP) was dangerous and would be the worst thing I could ever have done. Being rude to her would have got me killed, so the researchers have got us wrong. They don't know about us because we don't come forward, and we don't speak about this in therapy."

These study's findings highlight the unique symptoms associated with the "specific phobia-severe parental alienation and abduction anxiety variant" (Price-Tobler, 2023), which deviate from the previously described symptoms in earlier research. This discrepancy in symptom presentation adds to the growing understanding of different manifestations within the realm of specific phobia, anxiety, and abduction, underscoring the need for further research and exploration.

In addition, these studies report that children and adults exposed to SPAA who have experienced the new anxiety and abduction variant may still experience symptoms such as paranoia and phobia as adults. Furthermore, survivors report that due to the traumatic experience of being abducted by their AP and the brainwashing accompanying this act, as adults, they may still harbour a mild irrational fear of the TP (that they can withstand with therapy over time). However, the survivors report that their fear may turn into an intense, phobic fear of the AP adults. Finally, please note that the group of survivors within this study have all reconnected with their TP as part of the study criteria, and it is relevant at this stage to remind the reader due to the following information:

SPAA survivors in these studies reported that they are not as scared of their TP anymore but are very scared of what their APs can still do to them as adults. Many SPA and SPAA survivors stated that they still feel programmed by the AP, and it never stops. Consequently, the survivor may still be experiencing a range of symptoms from feeling enmeshed, not having a sense of self, no 'voice', paranoid thoughts, terror, withdrawal, selected mutism, cowering, or subservience. In addition, unsubstantiated theories, and beliefs that they are being watched or followed or may be killed by their TP or the TPs family or friends may still be running within their internal thought patterns.

These studies report that during the interviews, survivors identified their APs as still experiencing fluctuating bouts of persecutory delusion well into the APs' older ages. The Researcher hypothesises that these PABs do not stop due to the reenactment of the APs' cyclical maladaptive patterns. These studies also report that survivors describe a lifelong, unresolved, and unrelenting pattern that contributes to their heightened anxiety and distress, leading to difficulty functioning in everyday life. Fears and phobias experienced by survivors relating to harm as children can be very real to the client and must not be questioned or denied by MHPs. These are CITs that MHPs need to be sensitive, empathetic, and highly knowledgeable about, which is another reason why a specific treatment protocol urgently needs to be implemented.

SPAA and Factitious Disorder Imposed on Another

Building upon these observations, the Researcher further suggests that survivors of SPAA in these studies may have been exposed to a parent who actively engaged in psychological (shared delusions) or physical abuse toward them, a phenomenon known as factitious disorder imposed on another (FDIOA). This form of CIT involves the deliberate exaggeration or fabrication of a child's physical or psychological condition with the intention to deceive (American Psychiatric Association, 2013).

The Researcher reports a notable gap in the current knowledge regarding the association between survivors of SPAA and FDIOA and recommends that it is important to recognise that FDIOA extends beyond the mere fabrication of medical conditions or the insistence on a specific psychological diagnosis like autism. While FDIOA is commonly understood to showcase physical symptom presentations, it is crucial to acknowledge that psychological harm inflicted by APs on their children is also a significant CIT if the criteria for an FDIOA diagnosis are met. These studies report that the survivors of SPAA may still be under the invocation of FDIOA, and further research needs to be developed.

Continuing the quest for more information, the Researcher located the description of FDIOA within DSM-IV-TR, which was ambiguous and listed in the appendix as a condition requiring further investigation. However, within the DSM-5, it is also known as FDIOA and has been unambiguously described as a mental disorder (Hamilton & Kouchi, 2018). Understanding the dynamics of shared delusional disorders becomes essential in comprehending the experiences of survivors exposed to FDIOA. In addition, it highlights the potential for these individuals to have inherited or internalised the delusional beliefs imposed upon them during their upbringing, as described in these studies. Such insights contribute to a more comprehensive understanding of the psychological impact on survivors and the complexities of their CITs and lived experiences.

Building upon this description, the Researcher argues that these studies suggest that MHPs need to observe symptoms for FDIOA that may also link to the "specific phobia-severe parental alienation, and abduction anxiety variant" (Price-Tobler, 2023). After reading the DSM-5 criteria for FDIA, this conclusion was drawn as follows:

Criterion A involves falsifying psychological signs or symptoms or inducing an injury or disease in another, associated with identified deception (American Psychiatric Association, 2013). For example, previous research describes APs in the ABPA severe category as experiencing persecutory delusions (Childress, 2015). Furthermore, these studies report that survivors of SPAA were told delusional stories by their AP that they would be sexually abused, abducted, kidnapped, or killed by their TP. These studies report that the AP may still speak these abuse narratives even when the child becomes an adult. Criterion B states that the AP may present the child or adult survivor as a victim who has been impaired, ill, or injured to others. For example, one survivor spoke about their AP telling their friends about how sick the child was (and later as an adult-child) and how much they (the AP) bragged about being relied on when (as a child) they were not actually feeling sick.

Criterion C highlights that the deceptive behaviour by the AP is present and evident even when there are no obvious external rewards, such as needing money or compelling external incentives (Hamilton & Kouchi, 2018) from others. Criterion D specifies that a different mental disorder, such as a psychotic disorder, cannot explain the APs' behaviour. Finally, criterion E describes how some APs experience recurrent episodes where two or more falsified events of illness or induction of injury have been present. For example, survivors report that many APs are still trying to get them to believe their false stories of abuse as adults on every occasion that is presented.

These studies report that the severity and duration of these symptoms can manifest into adulthood and may vary based on individual circumstances. MHPs and mental health professionals may need to provide specialised support and intervention to help children and adult survivors to cope with these challenging, ongoing, relentless experiences. By recognising the 'specific phobia-severe parental alienation and abduction anxiety variant' (Price-Tobler, 2023) and the potential CIT of FDIOA, MHPs and other professionals working with child and adult survivors can provide more targeted and effective support. This Researcher stresses the importance of identifying different CITs and SPA variants to understand better and address the distinct impacts of childhood trauma on survivors.

This research reports that none of the three adult survivor study participants has found any MHPs who have noticed or mentioned (to their knowledge) the 'specific phobia anxiety variant' (Childress, 2015) symptoms or were able to identify where the indicators come from. The survivors also report that they have never recovered fully from their abuse. The survivors directly link these symptoms with suicidal ideation, explaining that the triggers are still invasive and can appear quickly when faced with someone who is an authoritative figure and is perceived to be trying to hurt them. For example, this can appear as a boss at work being too critical. The following extract is offered by "Alan", who experiences a 'specific phobia anxiety variant' (Childress, 2015) when he feels his nervous system dysregulate;

> We'll use this analogy – instead of the pictures being put into a photo album, the picture is always there. Any trigger, any time a situation reminds me of a trigger or reminds me of these pictures in my brain, bang, they are right there, right back again, I'm triggered, I'm in fight-flight-freeze – more freeze than anything else. It's when somebody's trying to get me to counter-transfer. Basically, anytime I don't feel safe, I lapse into starting to feel paranoid, and I just want to run. I get phobic about staying in an unsafe space. I have to leave. At that time, I feel suicidal, paranoid, and phobic. It's a bloody dangerous combination! I don't usually ever go back because I'm likely to kill myself when I'm in that point. (Interviewee Alan)

A second study participant who experienced SPAA with paranoia and anxiety since they were under five explained they had lived with these paranoid behaviours since being abducted by their mother and stepfather from her father's house one day by car. Once abducted, "Aurora" was moved into a boat offshore so no one could find her for a few weeks. "Aurora" was then flown by plane to the next destination. Consequently, the brainwashing and manipulation gradually escalated to a severe level as she became an adult, as described in the following extract;

> I carried my paranoia from being abducted well into adulthood. I wouldn't let my kids answer the door, I wouldn't answer the door, and I was always afraid – because we had these really fancy doors that are made of glass, and windows

> everywhere, and I wanted to block them out, but I didn't have the money to buy curtains, so I just got tinfoil and put them on the walls. I know it was a complete overreaction. I think that I was just so scared that someone would come and take me or my kids or that someone would be able to look in and see us while we're inside in the house. So, even watching scary movies where people were stalking and peeking in windows would set me off. I still do this even now, and I'm in my fifties. I didn't see my dad for forty-four years after the abduction. He died two years after we reunited. You can't tell me that taking kids away from their parent without consent isn't abduction. It is, and it stays with us forever. There's no recovery from abduction and severe parental alienation. It needs to be a criminal offence, but it isn't. (Interviewee Aurora)

Malingering by Proxy

Incorporating malingering by proxy as a facet of the study, the Researcher drew upon her professional experience working with adult survivors. Through her clinical practice, she observed instances of malingering by proxy and recognised its significance as another covert form of psychological manipulation within familial relationships. One example of malingering by proxy was when an AP was The decision to include malingering by proxy as a focus of investigation stemmed from the Researcher's commitment to comprehensively address the diverse range of complex trauma experiences encountered by adult survivors.

However, it is important to note that malingering by proxy was not initially part of the scope of the PhD study itself. Rather, it emerged from the Researcher's professional observations and insights gained from her work with adult survivors. Recognising the relevance of malingering by proxy as an additional covert tactic that may impact survivors' well-being, the Researcher sought to raise awareness of this phenomenon among MHPs.

For example, in the context of Malingering by Proxy, an AP may engage in a calculated scheme to withhold proper care for their child, all while exaggerating or fabricating their physical or psychological symptoms. The ultimate goal of this deceptive behaviour is to maintain financial benefits from organisations like Centrelink and the NDIS, which provide support based on the perceived level of care the child needs.

In this scenario, the AP may deliberately neglect the child's needs, such as medical appointments, educational support, or emotional nurturing, in order to portray them as more unwell than they truly are. By withholding essential care, the parent may create or exacerbate existing health issues, leading authorities to believe that the son requires more extensive support and resources than he does.

Furthermore, the AP may actively manipulate interactions with authorities or professionals involved in the son's care, providing misleading information or presenting exaggerated accounts of the child's condition to maintain the facade of necessity. This manipulation serves to reinforce the perception of the son as significantly impaired and deserving of continued financial assistance.

Overall, malingering by proxy in this context involves a calculated and deceptive strategy by the AP to exploit the son's perceived vulnerabilities for personal gain, ultimately at the expense of his well-being and development. It underscores the need for vigilant observation and thorough assessment by authorities and MHPs to identify and address such forms of psychological manipulation and abuse within familial relationships.

The inclusion of malingering by proxy in the broader discourse surrounding familial dynamics and psychological manipulation underscores the Researcher's dedication to equipping MHPs with a comprehensive understanding of trauma experiences. By bridging research and clinical practice, the Researcher aims to empower MHPs to effectively recognise and address the diverse manifestations of psychological abuse within familial relationships, ultimately enhancing the quality of care provided to adult survivors.

When an AP fabricates an illness in another person with the motivation that includes financial gain, avoiding work or family responsibilities, obtaining controlled narcotics, or manipulating legal proceedings, this is called Malingering by Proxy (Hamilton & Kouchi, 2018). It is important to note that "malingering" is not a psychiatric diagnosis per se, but it is included in the DSM-5 as a condition of clinical interest, identified by a "v" code (v65.2) (Hamilton & Kouchi, 2018). MHPs cannot diagnose FDIOA if there are strong external motivations that can explain why an AP would fabricate an illness in their child or adult survivor with the abovementioned motivations.

Cyberchondria

In addition to the aforementioned mental health conditions, an unexpected finding developed when the Researcher noticed an emerging phenomenon (namely cyberchondria) had been 'taught', as previously explained by Muris et al. (2002, p.1), to a survivor. The term "cyberchondria" describes excessive and repetitive online searching for personal health information, leading to distress, anxiety, and a loss of control over one's search behaviour (Newby & McElroy, 2020). Cyberchondria was reported by "Aurora" in these studies, and she reported knowing all about this topic. "Aurora" described her AP as teaching her cyberchondria behaviours that promoted her to search online for health-related subjects, which then turned into an addiction to finding medical answers.

Furthermore, this phenomenon is characterised by cognitive and affective aspects, including heightened concern about health and a pattern of repetitive and excessive online searches for health-related knowledge (Starcevic, 2017). The consequences of cyberchondria can be detrimental to survivors. Cyberchondria was investigated in a recent research study where 2,074 Chinese adolescent students (mean = 15.08 years, SD = 1.79) reported their demographic information, health anxiety, family dysfunction (divorce), optimism and cyberchondria (Liu et al., 2022).

Data from these studies suggest that survivors may have learnt cyberchondria symptoms and behaviours from their APs, and both the survivor and their AP may be displaying signs of cyberchondria well into their adult lives. Consequently, MHPs need to be looking out for symptomology in both the survivor and their AP. Furthermore, these studies report that research into the CITs between cyberchondria and SPA needs to be developed.

Persecutory Delusions After Abduction

As part of the broader investigation, it is crucial to examine the data concerning child abduction experiences and the persecutory delusions that survivors were exposed to by their APs. With the topic of suicidal ideation featured among the survivors of these studies, three participants also spoke about abduction healing and identity. Co-occurring examples of CITs of child maltreatment that survivors may have been exposed to include abduction, child kidnapping, child filicide, CSA, FDIOA, malingering by proxy, Stockholm syndrome, intergenerational cycles of trauma and violence, exploitation, and torture. The data gathered from these studies showed that one of the survivors was abducted and taken by car to a small plane by their mother and her new husband. This survivor also shared about her own continuous healing journey after the abduction and the need to straddle one world into a completely new and different world;

> I lived with my mother and father until I was abandoned by my mother at age three. I stayed living with my beloved father, but my mother and her new husband abducted me from my father at age five. Nobody helped me transition from that world into the new world and then how to accept the new world, and I remember thinking things like – I always

> wanted to go back. I never felt like this was my real world, and I always felt like I was a specimen in a fishbowl that – so to speak. The violent abuse toward me started right off the bat. I didn't have any kind of professional help in adapting to the change, to the drastic, very aggressive change. No one ever believed that I'd been abducted! So later on, when I was talking to my therapist, an identity crisis was revealed. I never was able to completely engage in that new world. I always had a foot in the other. I felt so relieved when she believed me! (Interviewee Aurora)

The second survivor also mentioned the theme of 'transitioning into a new world' after their interstate abduction and how he struggled with the aftereffects of being terrorised all his adult life psychologically;

> Always looking over your shoulder because we were taught that our father wasn't safe, that he was dangerous, and that he wanted to split us up. That was blatantly untrue, but how do you argue with someone who never allowed an argument in that space? They were the voice of God. Who were we to question that? We had no voice, we had no reason to disbelieve her, yet it was fuelled by her delusion that he was going to commit all these crimes to kidnap us, split us up, and we'd never see each other again, or anybody else in our family, when the reality of the situation was that was exactly what was happening to us by our mother! We were moved interstate covertly. He actually did know where we were because he had a mate who worked for the taxation department. What would he have done? What conversation would he have had with us that didn't terrify us and send us running? Because that's how we'd been conditioned. I always have that foot in another world and the other foot in this world ready to flee. How does a therapist work with that? (Interviewee Alan)

A third survivor who was abducted and taken internationally with their sibling by their father spoke of feeling abandoned once she and her sibling were taken by their father and how she literally had to fend for herself once abducted. These studies demonstrated that this participant showed dichotomous levels of emotion by combining the feelings of abandonment and luck at finding a new obsession after the abduction;

> Even though my dad took me away from my mum like it was international abduction. He kind of just abandoned me completely. And so, I became this child that had to sort of fend for itself, you know, and I was one of the lucky kids as my obsession was exercise. (Interviewee Antje-Renee)

Healing After Abduction

All three of the aforementioned participants in this chapter linked abduction with experiences of still struggling with what happened to them as adults and openly shared the impact of the highly fraught, forced transitions into a new world, not of their choosing or knowledge. The participants further shared in their interviews that they could also access MHPs who understood their stories and helped them move through parts of their SPA trauma during the foundation stages of healing and understanding.

Unfortunately, all three participants reported that they no longer see them privately. The two participants explained that they had outgrown their therapists (as they didn't know about SPA), and the other therapist who helped with childhood trauma, identity and abduction was not returning their calls to resume therapy, leaving two of the survivors reporting that they turn to the internet for education and healing for relief of individualised SPA symptoms. Unfortunately, all three participants also reported that these therapists were one of a long line of professionals who did not help.

Survivors who participated in these studies report that because of the lack of understanding among MH professionals regarding SPA education, survivors are turning to new ways to become empowered and begin their healing journey while waiting for MH professionals to catch up. The first participant turned to the internet for information on SPA due to a lack of knowledge among the MH professionals. This participant shared that she has started her healing journey, has grown a lot since accessing social media, and now feels strong enough to speak at parental alienation conferences if she's asked to;

> Healing. I'm healing, which is an action, so it's constant. Constantly taking action to work through these things better than I would have before. I know that I am important now, and whereas that was something I didn't grow up believing, especially after the abduction. So that was a huge shift in my beliefs and my mindset that I could be validated, and therapists can believe me, and my story is real, that it wasn't all made up and a joke. It wasn't something to laugh about. Suicide isn't so present with me these days, and I felt that I outgrew my last therapist and left. I've tried to see her again, but she isn't returning my calls, so I research SPA myself now on the internet, and I've learnt so much that I now speak at conferences when someone wants an adult survivor of SPA to share their story. I'm waiting for the therapists to catch up to me! (Interviewee Aurora)

A second participant shared that information gleaned from the internet has positively affected his personal SPA education level. How much he enjoys the information he learns is also revealed.

> There's a woman on Facebook. She's a holistic psychologist. She has a lot of insightful bits and pieces that she posts up. She's all about healing from parental trauma. She talks about,

> "Did you have a parent who did this? Did you have a parent who did that?" I find her work really helpful, and it resonates with me a lot. So that's one resource that I found. Some of the YouTube videos made by a clinical psychologist talk about the presence of this pathogen in relationships and in families and talk about alienation. I found some of his stuff was just gold. (Interviewee Alan)

The findings from these studies provide additional evidence for the recommendation that trauma research should incorporate lived experience researchers. Specifically, the discovery that a lived experience Researcher Practitioner has encountered similar accounts to her own from other survivors that have not been documented previously is equivalent to locating a needle in a haystack. This finding supports and aligns with the motto of SPA survivors, "nothing about us without us," which emphasises the importance of including the voices of survivors in trauma research about themselves (Price-Tobler, 2023). This approach addresses the historical absence of survivor perspectives in previous PA research and underscores the value of lived experience researchers in trauma research.

Furthermore, the Researcher puts forward another possible explanation for the lack of information on the topic of SPA and its variants. It is suggested that one reason for this gap may be the strong considerations that need to be put in place when researching children with anxiety sensitivity (Chorpita et al., 2010), combined with the ethical challenges of conducting interviews with young children who have undergone such traumatic experiences. For example, anxiety sensitivity is a construct that involves pairing interoceptive stimuli with adverse outcomes through interoceptive conditioning, observational learning, or the internalisation of rules or beliefs. This association is not typical among younger children, who often experience fear in response to the actual presence of a frightening or negative stimulus.

According to Piagetian theory, children in the concrete operational period of intellectual development (ages 7 to 11) may lack the cognitive ability to link internal sensations with future-oriented, abstract forms of danger, such as death, embarrassment, or losing one's mind. Thus, it is unlikely that they can differentiate the immediate discomfort of unpleasant sensations from their potential concerns. Consequently, an instrument like the Childhood Anxiety Sensitivity Index may lack utility in this age group when researching children experiencing SPAA at a young age, especially in children under eight. However, this is where the survivors can add their valuable contributions to the research because now, they report on previous childhood trauma that researchers can unravel, especially now as adults who have thought about the events from a more mature point of view.

Specific fears in young children can persist and carry on into adulthood (Muris et al., 2002), as described by many survivors in these studies. In addition, these studies report that specific fears and phobias have interfered with their normal functioning for their whole lives. Previous research has stated that children's fears and phobias are usually taught, whereas others report that these phenomena reflect "instinctual, spontaneous reactions to evolutionary prepotent cues" (Muris et al., 2002, p.1). Rachman (1977) reports that specific fears have three pathways regarding learning experiences that contribute to the acquisition of phobias and fears: 1. "aversive classical conditioning", 2. "modelling", and 3. "negative information transmission" (Muris et al., 2002, p.186).

In the context of SPAA, other learning experiences may also be relevant. For example, Chorpita and Barlow's (1998) work applies to this issue. They propose that early experiences with uncontrollable events could be considered a core pathway to the development of fear and anxiety because such experiences may increase the likelihood of perceiving events as beyond one's control (i.e., a "psychological vulnerability") (Muris et al., 2002, p.2). Furthermore, children raised with a sense of control have greater access to information that predicts the possibility of avoiding negative consequences, such as learning breech and repair sequencing (Childress, 2015). In contrast, children who experience a lack of control during development tend to store information that predicts that negative outcomes cannot be prevented. This information storage can lead to a decreased sense of control over events, increasing the likelihood of experiencing fear and anxiety in adulthood. As a result, further research is needed to investigate the specific phobia and anxiety variants identified in these studies.

Potential New Discovery Found Due to Being a Lived Experience Researcher

The findings from these studies emphasise the value of including lived experience researchers in trauma research. Particularly noteworthy is the potential discovery by a lived experience researcher and MHP of a new variety of specific phobia, which resonated with similar accounts from other survivors of severe parental alienation and abduction (SPAA). This finding underscores the importance of incorporating diverse perspectives, including those of individuals who have personally experienced trauma, to uncover nuances and phenomena that may have previously gone unrecognised by non-lived experience researchers.

Furthermore, the researcher reports that none of the three adult survivor study participants has found any MHPs who have ever noticed the 'specific phobia' (Childress, 2015) symptoms or were able to identify where the symptoms developed from. The survivors also report that they have never recovered from this new variant. The survivors directly link these symptoms with suicidal ideation, explaining that the triggers are still invasive and can appear quickly at any time they are faced with someone who is an authoritative figure and is perceived to be trying to hurt them. This can appear in the form of a boss at work being too critical. The following extract is offered by "Alan", who experiences 'specific phobia' (Childress, 2015) when he feels his nervous system dysregulate;

> We'll use this analogy – instead of the pictures being put into a photo album, the picture is always there. Any trigger, any time a situation reminds me of a trigger or reminds me of these pictures in my brain, bang, they are right there, right back again, I'm triggered, I'm in fight-flight-freeze – more freeze than anything else. It's when somebody's trying to get me to counter-transfer. Basically, anytime I don't feel safe, I lapse into starting to feel paranoid, and I just want to run. I get phobic about staying in an unsafe space. I have to leave. At that time, I feel suicidal, paranoid, and phobic. It's a bloody dangerous combination! I don't usually ever go back because I'm likely to kill myself when I'm in that point. (Interviewee Alan)

A second study participant who experienced what they believed to be the new "phobia and paranoia due to specific phobia-anxiety variant" since they were under five explained they had lived with these paranoid behaviours since being abducted by their mother and stepfather from her father's house one day by car. Once abducted, "Aurora" was moved into a boat offshore so no one could find her for a few weeks. "Aurora" was then flown by plane to the next destination. Consequently, the brain-washing and manipulation gradually escalated to a severe level as an adult, as described in the following extract;

I carried my paranoia from being abducted well into adulthood. I wouldn't let my kids answer the door, I wouldn't answer the door, and I was always afraid – because we had these really fancy doors that are made of glass, and windows everywhere, and I wanted to block them out, but I didn't have the money to buy curtains, so I just got tinfoil and put them on the walls. I know it was a complete overreaction. I think that I was just so scared that someone would come and take me or my kids or that someone would be able to look in and see us while we're inside in the house. So even watching scary movies where people were stalking and peeking in windows would set me off. I still do this even now, and I'm in my fifties. I didn't see my dad for forty-four years after the abduction. He died two years after we reunited. You can't tell me that taking kids away from their parent without consent isn't abduction. It is, and it stays with us forever. There's no recovery from abduction and severe parental alienation. It needs to be a criminal offence, but it isn't. (Interviewee Aurora)

Exploring Complex Intersecting Traumas Post-Thesis

Complex intersecting traumas (CITs) encompass a range of intertwined experiences that individuals endure across their lifespan, particularly in the context of childhood psychological abuse persisting into adulthood. These traumas, including parental alienation, emotional abuse, physical abuse, sexual abuse, neglect, traumatic family dynamics, social isolation, stigmatisation, and interpersonal betrayal, coalesce to create multifaceted challenges for survivors and the MHPs who work with them.

Please note: The following inclusion of additional post-doctoral research from the PhD enriches and augments the original findings presented in the thesis. Integrating this supplementary data makes the research more comprehensive and provides a deeper understanding of the subject matter. This extra research allows for further exploration of the topic, addressing any gaps or unanswered questions from the original study. Additionally, it enhances the utility of the PhD by offering updated information, new insights, and expanded analyses, which can be invaluable for mental health practitioners, researchers, and other stakeholders in the field. The original thesis content continues in Theme Four.

Characterised by chronic stress, instability, and profound emotional distress, these experiences often manifest in symptoms of post-traumatic stress disorder (PTSD), depression, anxiety, disordered eating, substance abuse, self-harm, and difficulties in forming and maintaining relationships. Despite the unique manifestations of each trauma, their cumulative and synergistic effects exacerbate the overall impact, complicating the healing process for adult survivors.

Addressing CITs necessitates a comprehensive and holistic approach to therapy, incorporating trauma-informed care, psychoeducation, support groups, self-care practices, and the cultivation of validating relationships. By recognising the nuanced experiences of survivors and providing them with tailored support and resources, MHPs can facilitate their journey toward healing, resilience, and empowerment. MHPs play a crucial role in supporting adult survivors of PA on their journey of self-discovery and healing.

These survivors often carry deep emotional wounds from their experiences, struggling to understand themselves and embrace their true identity fully. Without guidance and support, they may continue to grapple with feelings of inadequacy, self-doubt, and a pervasive sense of disconnection from themselves and others. By helping adult survivors explore and embrace their unique quirks, idiosyncrasies, and perceived imperfections, MHPs empower them to reclaim their sense of self-worth and confidence. Through compassionate guidance and reflection, therapists can assist survivors in recognising the value of their individuality and the richness it brings to their lives.

Furthermore, MHPs can help survivors navigate the challenges of self-acceptance and authenticity, providing a safe space for them to explore their innermost thoughts, feelings, and experiences. By fostering a supportive therapeutic environment, MHPs encourage survivors to let go of their defences and embrace vulnerability, paving the way for profound personal growth and healing.

Ultimately, MHPs have the opportunity to help adult survivors cultivate a deeper understanding of themselves, their strengths, and their inherent worthiness. Through this transformative process, survivors can break free from the shackles of PA abuse and embark on a journey toward self-discovery, empowerment, and genuine connection with themselves and others. Practitioners should be vigilant for complex intersecting traumas in adult survivors because they can significantly impact the individual's well-being and mental health. By understanding and addressing these traumas, MHPs can provide more effective and tailored support to the survivors.

Identifying and acknowledging these traumas can help validate the survivor's experiences and feelings, fostering a sense of understanding and empathy. This validation is crucial for the survivor's healing process and can contribute to rebuilding their sense of self-worth and empowerment. Moreover, recognising the complex interplay between different traumas allows practitioners to develop comprehensive treatment plans that address the multiple layers of the survivor's experiences. This holistic approach can lead to more successful outcomes and better long-term recovery.

The content of this book, which encompasses interviews with adult survivors (as described previously) as well as various examples of potential CITs experienced by survivors of child psychological abuse, serves as a valuable resource for survivors and MHPs. It provides insight into the diverse range of traumas and challenges survivors face, helping practitioners tailor their interventions to address specific needs and concerns. The following are just a few examples from the extensive collection of incidents that have been documented, which will be published in a forthcoming book due to space constraints. Additionally, it can guide practitioners in recognising patterns of abuse and manipulation perpetrated by APs, facilitating more informed and targeted interventions.

Limited Understanding of Heritage and Identity

Adult survivors may have a limited understanding of their heritage and identity due to restricted access to information from the TPs side of the family. This reliance on the AP for identity formation can further perpetuate control and manipulation. This limited understanding of heritage and identity can significantly impact adult survivors, depriving them of a crucial aspect of their sense of self. Without access to information from the TPs side of the family, survivors may struggle to piece together their familial history and cultural background.

This reliance on the AP for identity formation can further perpetuate control and manipulation, as the AP may selectively provide or distort information to suit their agenda. As a result, survivors may grapple with feelings of disconnection from their roots, uncertainty about their cultural identity, and a sense of incompleteness in understanding their heritage. This lack of clarity and connection to their familial past can contribute to ongoing emotional distress and identity struggles in adulthood. Additionally, relying solely on the AP for identity formation can perpetuate control and manipulation. The AP may selectively provide or distort information to suit their agenda, leaving survivors with a skewed or incomplete understanding of their heritage.

Unresolved Traumas Projected onto Survivors From their AP

This pattern is concerning because it perpetuates a cycle of emotional manipulation and psychological distress. When adult survivors devote significant energy to identifying unresolved traumas projected onto them by the AP, they become enmeshed in a dynamic that prioritises the AP's needs and emotions over their own well-being. This process can lead to feelings of guilt, self-doubt, and confusion as survivors internalise the AP's narratives and struggle to differentiate their own experiences from those imposed upon them.

Additionally, focusing excessively on the AP's unresolved traumas detracts from survivors' ability to address their own healing and personal growth. It reinforces a sense of dependency on the AP's emotional state and perpetuates patterns of co-dependency and emotional enmeshment. Ultimately, this dynamic hinders survivors' ability to establish healthy boundaries, develop autonomy, and cultivate a strong sense of self.

Survivor Taught to Alienate Others

This behaviour is detrimental because it perpetuates a cycle of abuse and perpetuates the harmful effects of PA across generations. When survivors are taught to alienate others, including their own children and grandchildren, they become complicit in continuing the pattern of emotional manipulation and psychological harm that they themselves experienced. By alienating their own offspring, survivors not only perpetuate the trauma they endured but also inflict similar pain and suffering on their offspring. This behaviour creates a toxic family dynamic characterised by fractured relationships, emotional turmoil, and long-term psychological damage for both the survivor and the subsequent generations. It reinforces harmful beliefs and behaviours learned from their AP, further entrenching the cycle of abuse and making it difficult to break free from its grip.

Additionally, alienating others can isolate the survivor from potential sources of support and healing, exacerbating their feelings of loneliness, guilt, and shame. Overall, this pattern of behaviour contributes to the intergenerational transmission of trauma and undermines the survivor's ability to break free from the cycle of abuse.

Gaslighting and Confusion of Memories

Gaslighting by APs can be detrimental as it leads to the manipulation and distortion of childhood memories and experiences for adult survivors. This can result in confusion, self-doubt, and a distorted perception of reality, making it difficult for survivors to trust their own memories and perceptions. It undermines their sense of self and can contribute to ongoing psychological distress and emotional instability.

Grief and Primal Loss

Grief and the primal loss of a TP can deeply affect survivors, impacting their emotional well-being and sense of identity. The loss of family connections and relationships due to PA can lead to profound feelings of loneliness, abandonment, and disconnection. These experiences may exacerbate feelings of loss and longing for the love and support that their family should have provided. Additionally, unresolved grief and primal loss can contribute to ongoing emotional struggles and difficulties in forming healthy relationships in adulthood.

Manipulative Behaviour and Domestic Conflict

Survivors often find themselves entangled in domestic conflicts orchestrated by their APs, leading to emotional distress and potential legal intervention to mediate disputes. Manipulative behaviour and domestic conflict such as family and domestic violence between family members, orchestrated by APs are detrimental to the well-being of survivors, exacerbating their trauma and emotional distress. By engaging in manipulative tactics, APs create a toxic family environment characterised by ongoing tension and potential apprehended violence orders. This manipulation undermines the survivor's sense of security and stability, leaving them feeling trapped in a cycle of emotional turmoil. Moreover, the conflict instigated by APs complicates legal matters, forcing survivors to navigate legal interventions to resolve disputes within the family. As a result, survivors experience heightened levels of stress and anxiety, impeding their ability to heal and move forward in their recovery journey. Ultimately, manipulative behaviour perpetuates the cycle of abuse, hindering survivors from breaking free and reclaiming their autonomy and emotional well-being.

Intimate Partner and Family and Domestic Violence

Survivors, accustomed to such behaviours due to their upbringing in environments marred by PA, often struggle to recognise the abusive nature of their relationships, making it challenging for MHPs to intervene effectively. As a result, it becomes crucial for MHPs to possess a deep understanding of FDV dynamics to effectively support survivors in recognising and addressing these harmful patterns, facilitating their journey towards healing and empowerment.

Parental Suicides and Threats

Additionally, AP may have used threats of self-harm or suicide to manipulate and control the survivor, leading to feelings of guilt and responsibility. This is harmful because it places undue emotional burden and responsibility on the survivor, leading to feelings of guilt, anxiety, and helplessness. When an AP threatens self-harm or suicide as a means of manipulation and control, it creates a toxic dynamic where the survivor feels responsible for the AP's well-being and safety. This emotional manipulation can lead to a sense of powerlessness and emotional distress for the survivors as they struggle to navigate the guilt and fear associated with the AP's threats. Additionally, it undermines the survivor's sense of autonomy and agency, as they may feel compelled to comply with the AP's demands out of fear of the consequences.

Emotional Incest and Parentification

Survivors may have experienced emotional incest and parentification, blurring boundaries and perpetuating dysfunctional relationship dynamics. Emotional incest and parentification are harmful because they disrupt the natural boundaries and roles within the parent-child relationship, leading to emotional and psychological distress for the survivor. Emotional incest involves the inappropriate emotional involvement or dependency of a child by a parent, where the parent relies on the child for emotional support or validation that peers or other adults should provide. This blurring of boundaries can create confusion and a sense of betrayal for the survivor, as they may feel overwhelmed by the parent's emotional demands.

Parentification occurs when a child is forced into caregiving or responsibility for the parent or other siblings, assuming adult-like responsibilities at a young age. This can lead to the suppression of the child's own needs and desires, as well as a loss of childhood innocence and autonomy. Parentification also perpetuates dysfunctional relationship dynamics, as the child may struggle to assert their own identity and develop healthy boundaries in future relationships.

Navigating Self-Harm and Mental Health Challenges

Survivors may engage in self-harm behaviours combined with mental health issues such as anxiety, depression, eating disorders, and substance abuse (to name a few) as a result of the trauma endured. Engaging in self-harm behaviours and experiencing mental health challenges are detrimental because they indicate significant psychological distress and suffering for the survivor. These behaviours and conditions often serve as coping mechanisms to manage overwhelming emotions and trauma-related symptoms but ultimately exacerbate the survivor's suffering and increase their risk of further harm.

Self-harm behaviours, such as cutting or burning oneself, are maladaptive coping strategies that provide temporary relief from emotional pain but can lead to serious physical injuries and long-term health consequences. They also perpetuate feelings of shame, guilt, and self-loathing, reinforcing negative self-perceptions and low self-worth.

Mental health issues such as depression and anxiety can significantly impair the survivor's daily functioning, affecting their ability to maintain relationships, work, and engage in activities they once enjoyed. These conditions often co-occur with trauma-related symptoms such as hypervigilance, flashbacks, and intrusive memories, further complicating the survivor's recovery process.

Furthermore, eating disorders and substance abuse may develop as ways to cope with underlying emotional pain and distress. Still, they can lead to severe physical health complications and increase the risk of addiction and overdose. These behaviours also contribute to a cycle of self-destructive patterns and exacerbate feelings of hopelessness and despair.

Exposure to Familicide and Familicide- Threats

Survivors may have witnessed or been threatened with family homicide or attempted homicide by the AP, leading to trauma and fear. Exposure to familicide or threats of familicide by the AP is deeply distressing and harmful to the survivor's psychological well-being for several reasons. First and foremost, witnessing or being threatened with such extreme violence within the family context creates profound trauma and fear, often resulting in long-lasting emotional scars and psychological distress.

Familicide, the intentional killing of one's own family members, represents the ultimate betrayal of trust and safety within the family unit. Survivors who witness or are threatened with familicide may experience overwhelming feelings of terror, helplessness, and powerlessness as they are confronted with the potential loss of their loved ones and their own lives.

Moreover, exposure to familicide or threats of familicide shatters the survivor's sense of security and stability, leaving them constantly on edge and hypervigilant for signs of danger. The trauma associated with such events can manifest in various ways, including nightmares, flashbacks, anxiety, and avoidance behaviours, which disrupt the survivor's ability to function in daily life and maintain healthy relationships.

Violence and Torture

Survivors may have endured direct threats of violence and torture from family members or experienced such acts firsthand. Additionally, they might have witnessed their siblings or parents undergoing torture. Exposure to threats of violence and torture, whether experienced firsthand or witnessed within the family, has profound and lasting negative effects on survivors' mental and emotional well-being.

Firstly, such experiences instil deep-seated fear and anxiety in survivors, leading to ongoing psychological distress and trauma. The constant threat of violence creates a pervasive sense of insecurity and vulnerability, making it difficult for survivors to feel safe in their environment or relationships with others.

Secondly, witnessing or experiencing violence and torture can shatter survivors' trust in familial relationships and authority figures. It erodes the sense of safety and protection that should be inherent within the family unit, leaving survivors feeling abandoned, betrayed, and alone. Moreover, exposure to violence and torture can have long-lasting impacts on survivors' physical health, exacerbating existing health conditions or leading to the development of new ones. Chronic stress and trauma from such experiences can contribute to a range of physical ailments, including cardiovascular problems, gastrointestinal issues, and immune system disorders.

Additionally, survivors may struggle with profound feelings of guilt, shame, and self-blame as they grapple with the aftermath of violence and torture. They may internalise the belief that they somehow deserved or provoked the abuse, further undermining their self-worth and contributing to ongoing mental health challenges. Furthermore, the emotional scars left by exposure to violence and torture can impair survivors' ability to form healthy relationships, regulate their emotions, and navigate daily life. They may experience difficulties trusting others, managing stress, and coping with adversity, which can impact their functioning in various domains, including work, education, and social interactions.

Exposure to Gun Violence and Traumatic Loss

Survivors may also have witnessed gun violence within their homes or communities, resulting in traumatic experiences and thoughts of self-harm. Adult survivors may have had APs who were involved in criminal activities or surrounded by questionable individuals, which may have posed a heightened risk to the survivor's safety. They may also have been hurt by these individuals or may have been coerced into illegal activities themselves.

In cases involving a gang, the repercussions could be even more severe. The survivor may have faced direct threats or violence from gang members, leading to heightened fear and trauma. Additionally, they may have been coerced into criminal activities or forced to maintain silence about the gang's actions, further complicating their situation and perpetuating feelings of powerlessness.

Furthermore, APs may have instigated the disappearance or death of a TP, perpetuating a profound sense of loss and abandonment for survivors, grappling with unresolved grief and emotional turmoil, and fostering ongoing cycles of trauma and instability, especially amid ongoing criminal investigations.

Substance Abuse and Introduction to Drugs

Survivors may have been introduced to drugs and alcohol by their APs as a means of control or manipulation. The exposure of survivors to substance abuse, particularly by APs in addiction, often serves as a tool for control or manipulation within the family dynamic. For instance, some survivors recall cases where they were introduced to drugs or alcohol by their parents as a form of reward or incentive for compliance. For example, one participant recounted how their TP offered them alcohol as a reward for keeping her company, highlighting the harmful effects of parental substance abuse on children's upbringing and well-being.

Drugging Child and Adolescent Survivors

Drugging a child or adolescent survivor may have served various purposes beyond ensuring quietness. In some cases, parents may use drugs to control or manipulate the behaviour of their offspring, making them more compliant or easier to manage. Additionally, drugs might have been used as a form of punishment or to induce sleep, giving the parent a sense of control over the household dynamics. Moreover, in situations involving substance abuse issues within the family, parents may inadvertently or purposefully expose their offspring to drugs or alcohol, leading to long-term psychological and physical consequences.

Compulsive Lying and Normalisation of Abuse

Some survivors may exhibit compulsive lying behaviours, possibly learned from observing their APs' deceptive actions. This behaviour perpetuates a cycle of deceit and undermines trust within relationships. Compulsive lying, often learned from observing the deceptive actions of APs, becomes normalised as a means of navigating conflict and asserting control. It reflects a deficiency in healthy conflict resolution skills and autonomy, serving as a coping mechanism for anxiety and internalised trauma. Ultimately, it reinforces a distorted perception of reality and inhibits genuine emotional connections, posing significant challenges to the survivor's interpersonal relationships and overall well-being. This behaviour may stem from a lack of healthy conflict resolution skills and maybe a coping mechanism for anxiety and limited autonomy.

Coercive Adoption Tactics: Alienation's Impact on Parental Bonds

This type of manipulation is driven by the AP's desire to solidify their control over the child and erase any semblance of connection with the TP. By convincing the child that the TP does not love them and encouraging adoption by the stepparent, the AP seeks to sever the child's ties to their biological parent and replace them with a new caregiver who is more aligned with their interests. This tactic exploits the child's vulnerability and desire for love and stability, coercing them into accepting the stepparent as a substitute for the TP. Ultimately, it serves to reinforce the AP's authority and diminish the child's sense of identity and autonomy.

Exploring Sexual Abuse by Associates of AP

Survivors reported instances where the partner or associates of the AP had harmed them. Additionally, the AP may have been aware of these incidents but opted not to act due to disbelief, fear of community judgment, or concern over the stability of their relationship. This delayed reporting can further endanger the survivor and perpetuate cycles of abuse. Furthermore, child and adult survivors may have experienced being spied on by a step-parent, partner, or acquaintance of the AP, which can exacerbate the emotional trauma and psychological distress experienced by the child.

When a child is subjected to surveillance without their knowledge or consent, it violates their sense of privacy and autonomy. This intrusion into their personal space can further erode the child's trust and security, exacerbating feelings of vulnerability and isolation. Moreover, if the spying is conducted with malicious intent or used to manipulate or control the child, it can perpetuate the cycle of abuse inherent in child psychological abuse. Overall, such actions can have profound and long-lasting effects on the child's emotional well-being and development, perpetuating the harmful dynamics of SPA and exacerbating the child's sense of betrayal and loss.

Disclosure of Sexual abuse to AP by a Step-parent, Friend, or Family Member

Survivors of child psychological abuse may encounter significant challenges when disclosing their experiences, particularly if the perpetrator holds a position of authority or trust within the family. Accusations from both the abuser and the AP can further complicate the situation, leading to disbelief or scepticism from other family members unwilling to confront the issue. This dynamic may perpetuate a cycle of abuse, as the perpetrator may retaliate against the survivor to maintain control and silence them, exacerbating the survivor's emotional turmoil and distress. Fear of repercussions and uncertainty about how others will receive their disclosure can further isolate the survivor within their family or social circle, creating additional barriers to seeking help.

Moreover, disclosing abuse may trigger legal proceedings or involvement from child protective services, adding another layer of stress and trauma for the survivor. The prospect of legal action can intensify feelings of vulnerability and anxiety, particularly if the survivor anticipates backlash or resistance from those close to the perpetrator. Despite the potential for conflict or disruption within familial and social relationships, survivors must navigate the complex process of disclosure to access the support and protection they desperately need.

Impact on Survivor if APs Relationship Ends

When an APs relationship faces turmoil or dissolution, they may unleash their frustration and anger upon the survivor, especially if the survivor does not align with their wishes or desires. This retaliation can take various forms, ranging from verbal abuse to punitive actions to exert control and punishment. The survivor may become a target for the AP's pent-up emotions and insecurities, leading to a cycle of emotional distress and instability within the family dynamic.

In instances of relationship breakdowns, the AP's need for control intensifies, often resulting in heightened levels of manipulation and coercion directed towards the survivor. This can manifest in punitive measures, such as restricting access to resources, isolating the survivor from support networks, or inflicting psychological harm. As the survivor refuses to conform to the AP's expectations or challenges their authority, the AP's punitive behaviours may escalate, further exacerbating the survivor's feelings of fear, helplessness, and isolation.

Additionally, APs may resort to extreme measures, such as destroying or burning the survivor's cherished personal belongings, as a means of exerting dominance and instilling fear in the survivor. Furthermore, they may punish survivors by removing basic necessities such as hot water, heating, and adequate food. Additionally, some APs have gone as far as harming, killing, or disposing of family pets as a means of further isolating and punishing the survivor.

Technology-Facilitated Abuse and Coercive Control

Adult survivors may experience technology-facilitated abuse, where the AP uses drones, tracking devices or spying apps to monitor their whereabouts, texts, calls, and social media activities. This form of abuse is invasive in nature, and the erosion of privacy and autonomy it inflicts upon the survivor. By utilising technology to monitor every aspect of the survivor's life, including their movements, communications, and online interactions, the AP establishes an insidious form of control that can be suffocating and oppressive.

For survivors with disabilities or mental health challenges, this type of coercion can be especially damaging, as it further exacerbates feelings of vulnerability and powerlessness. Additionally, technology-facilitated abuse can have long-lasting psychological effects, instilling a sense of constant surveillance and fear in the survivor, even after they have escaped the abusive situation. Overall, this manipulation of technology to perpetrate coercive control represents a grave violation of the survivor's rights and dignity, highlighting the urgent need for intervention and support.

Poverty and Single Parenthood

Survivors may face economic hardship within a single-parent household. Survivors may have been continuously exposed to a narrative that portrays their family as broken and inferior due to their AP's single-parent status, which can contribute to feelings of inadequacy and shame.

Moreover, survivors may experience ongoing comparisons between the TPs financial status and that of the AP, leading to feelings of resentment and injustice. This comparison is often compounded by the AP's manipulation tactics, such as withholding essential information about medical and school matters unless it serves their financial interests. This exploitation of the survivor's economic vulnerability and emotional well-being further perpetuates the cycle of control and manipulation, ultimately undermining their sense of agency and self-worth.

Thus, the combination of poverty and single parenthood resulting from the AP's potential alienation tactics represents a form of systemic abuse that inflicts both tangible and psychological harm on the survivor. The survivor may also have experienced reminders of the AP's sacrifices to provide for them. This creates a narrative of indebtedness, where the child feels obligated to show allegiance to the AP.

Parentification and Material Loss

Survivors may have been forced into parental roles, managing household affairs, or caring for siblings from a young age. This dynamic often arises due to parentification, where children are forced into adult roles prematurely, assuming responsibilities beyond their years. Additionally, survivors may have experienced significant material loss, such as the disappearance or destruction of personal belongings, which further compounds their burdens and sense of precocious maturity. "Precocious" in this context refers to an advanced level of maturity or development beyond what is considered typical for a person of that age.

Homelessness and Acts of Survival

Runaway and survival strategies by survivors often emerge as desperate attempts to escape abusive environments and navigate the tumultuous aftermath of SPA. Fleeing from abusive situations may force survivors into a precarious existence where they resort to substance abuse and risky behaviours as coping mechanisms. The need for immediate relief from emotional distress and the absence of stable support systems push survivors towards harmful survival strategies, further exacerbating their vulnerability and isolation.

Survivors may resort to engaging in challenging acts for survival, such as experiencing homelessness, turning to drug use, or engaging in sex work, as desperate measures to leave the dysfunctional household to cope with the trauma inflicted by the AP. These behaviours often stem from a deep sense of desperation and hopelessness, exacerbated by the emotional and psychological abuse endured within the family dynamic. The lack of familial support and the overwhelming burden of navigating life without a stable foundation can drive survivors to extreme measures in their quest for survival and emotional numbing.

In addition to resorting to desperate measures for survival, survivors may also seek solace and support by looking for a safe group of friends or peers on the street. This search for companionship and understanding stems from a fundamental human need for connection and validation, especially without a nurturing and supportive family environment. By finding solidarity and camaraderie among like-minded individuals, survivors hope to alleviate some of the isolation and alienation they experience as a result of their tumultuous upbringing. However, even within these social circles, survivors may still grapple with feelings of shame and inadequacy as the scars of their past trauma continue to influence their present interactions and relationships.

The Human Body as a Currency for Love

The practice of using bodies as currency for love reflects a profound distortion of healthy relationships and boundaries instilled by the AP. This manipulation fosters a toxic dynamic where survivors equate their worth with their ability to provide physical affection or gratification. As a result, some survivors may internalise the belief that their value lies solely in their capacity to fulfil the desires of others, perpetuating a cycle of exploitation and emotional deprivation.

In response to this dehumanising treatment, some survivors may opt for perpetual singledom as a means of reclaiming autonomy and shielding themselves from further exploitation. By eschewing romantic relationships, they seek to safeguard their physical and emotional well-being, refusing to participate in a system that devalues their intrinsic worth.

Addiction and Correctional Facilities

Within the confines of correctional facilities, survivors may have faced significant challenges related to addiction and endured trauma as a result of their incarceration. The structured environment of jail often exacerbates pre-existing substance abuse issues, leading survivors to grapple with withdrawal symptoms, cravings, and the allure of illicit substances within a constrained setting. Additionally, the inherent stress and power dynamics of prison life can contribute to the development or exacerbation of mental health disorders, further complicating the recovery process. Survivors may also be vulnerable to exploitation and victimisation by other inmates or staff members, compounding their trauma and sense of vulnerability. Moreover, the lack of adequate mental health and rehabilitation services within correctional facilities can perpetuate cycles of addiction and trauma, leaving survivors ill-equipped to address their underlying child abuse and reintegrate into society upon release.

Additionally, no specific studies have been performed on how many adult children of PA there are in the correctional facilities to the authors' knowledge. The specific number of children of divorce in the prison system can vary depending on various factors such as demographics, socioeconomic status, and individual circumstances. However, the Researcher suggests that children of divorced parents may be at a higher risk of experiencing adverse outcomes, including involvement in the criminal justice system, compared to those from intact families. Factors such as family instability, parental conflict, and disrupted family dynamics can contribute to increased delinquency and antisocial behaviour among children of divorce. While it's essential to recognise these risk factors, it's also crucial to approach the issue with nuance and consider the multitude of factors that can influence a child's trajectory. This area holds an opportunity for more research to be undertaken.

Survivors as Confidants- Parental Divorce Disclosure

Confiding in children during legal matters can be detrimental for several reasons. Firstly, it places undue emotional burden and responsibility on the child, forcing them to navigate complex legal situations for which they are ill-equipped. Children may feel overwhelmed, confused, and anxious as they grapple with adult issues beyond their comprehension, potentially leading to long-term psychological harm.

Additionally, involving children in legal proceedings can compromise their safety and well-being, exposing them to further risk of manipulation, coercion, or retribution from involved parties. Furthermore, confiding in children during legal matters undermines their right to a childhood free from adult concerns and responsibilities, depriving them of the opportunity to develop in a nurturing and supportive environment.

APs Changing Their Narrative

Changing one's story or narrative, especially to manipulate or deceive others, is unacceptable because it undermines truth and integrity. While trauma can indeed impact memory and perception, intentionally altering one's story for personal gain or to evade accountability is unethical and harmful. It perpetuates a cycle of dishonesty and erodes trust in relationships and institutions. Additionally, labelling such behaviour as acceptable due to trauma further normalises dishonesty and undermines efforts to address the root causes of the trauma. It's essential to promote honesty, accountability, and ethical behaviour in all aspects of life, especially in the context of interpersonal relationships and legal proceedings.

False Accusations of Family and Domestic Violence

Survivors may have been exposed to instances where the AP falsely accuses the TP of FDV. Additionally, the AP may repeat these accusations with subsequent partners, thus perpetuating a pattern of false allegations. Consequently, children and adolescents are taught that it is acceptable to make unfounded accusations to manipulate others and achieve personal objectives. This behaviour not only undermines the integrity of the legal system but also erodes trust and creates a toxic environment where dishonesty and manipulation are normalised.

Falsely accusing someone of FDV or manipulating accusations for personal gain is harmful and unjust. It undermines the seriousness of domestic violence, which is a severe form of abuse with significant legal and social implications. False accusations can tarnish the reputation and livelihood of innocent individuals, causing irreparable damage to their lives and relationships. Moreover, manipulating accusations of domestic violence to gain leverage or control in personal or legal matters perpetuates a cycle of abuse and further victimises genuine survivors of domestic violence. It erodes trust in the legal system and undermines efforts to support and protect victims of abuse.

Violent APs Masquerading as Fragile Victims- A Threat to Genuine Survivors

It is deeply concerning when individuals manipulate perceptions of FDV to portray themselves as victims when they are, in fact, the perpetrators. This behaviour not only obscures the truth but also undermines efforts to support genuine victims of domestic violence.

When an AP falsely presents themselves as a victim of domestic violence, it not only distorts the reality of the situation but also places genuine survivors at risk. By falsely portraying themselves as victims, these individuals may garner sympathy and support, making it more challenging for authorities to identify and intervene in cases of genuine abuse. The manipulation of FDV narratives by abusive individuals poses a significant threat to the feminist movement and undermines the plight of genuine victims. When perpetrators falsely portray themselves as victims, they distort reality and hinder efforts to support those in genuine need.

This deceptive behaviour not only obscures the truth but also endangers genuine survivors needing help. By garnering sympathy and support through false victimhood, perpetrators make it harder for authorities to identify and intervene in cases of actual abuse. Moreover, this manipulation perpetuates cycles of abuse within families, allowing the perpetrator to maintain control and continue their harmful behaviour unchecked. This hindrance in the fight against domestic violence is compounded by the fact that men can also be victims, highlighting the urgency of addressing this issue and ensuring justice for all involved parties.

It is crucial for MHPs and legal professionals to systematically investigate allegations of domestic violence and discern the truth, ensuring that genuine victims are protected and perpetrators are held accountable. Additionally, efforts must be made to raise awareness about the tactics used by manipulative individuals to falsely portray themselves as victims, thereby preventing further harm and ensuring justice for all parties involved.

KEY THEME FOUR (PHYSICAL HEALTH)

Survivors' Perspectives

Previous Physical Health Research

Previously undertaken research regarding the physical health manifestations experienced by survivors of child abuse and the CIT associations to SPA has been limited. Chapter One investigated prior research on this topic, reporting that adverse physical effects are the number one cause of death in adults who have experienced complex trauma as children (Felitti et al., 1998). Another study reporting on early traumatic events that survivors may have been exposed to describes the probability of an increased risk for physical health challenges such as asthma and heart disease (Perry, 2003).

The Researcher also located a further study reporting that cumulative toxic stress during a divorce crisis can have long-lasting adverse effects on children and has been shown to induce hypothalamic-pituitary-adrenal (HPA) and epigenetic changes, with consequent increases in reported rates of adult diseases, including stroke, heart disease, and diabetes (Kleinsorge & Covitz, 2012). Prolonged stress exposure has also been associated with developmental and cognitive delays that can adversely influence a child's linguistic, academic, and social functioning (Goldin & Salani, 2020). Lastly, epigenetic changes were also listed in previous research and are described as a phenomenon in gene expression that can arise from tumultuous environmental stimuli without a change in genotype (Gentner & O'Connor-Leppert, 2019).

Please note that questions regarding the participants' physical health were not asked as part of the study. However, due to the lack of research in the SPA area, all anomalous data from these studies were also deemed important and thoroughly analysed. Consequently, the Researcher noted any mention of physical diagnoses and symptoms experienced by survivors. Interestingly, six survivors reported their health conditions to the Researcher and then requested that their symptoms and diagnoses be included in these studies (during the interviews). The study participants requested that the Researcher include their biological health perspectives and explained that recording this data was important as they do not feel that medical doctors understand where their adverse health conditions develop from, hence why this anomalous data has been included.

Health Challenges

Interestingly, six participants mentioned 27 health challenges during the interview without being asked. For some participants, these symptoms started when they were young. For example, one male participant explained that he nearly died as a young person in a hospital and still suffers from ongoing related health challenges as an adult;

> As a child, I got MRSA and had to fight for my life because of the musty old chillin' on the hospital wall as if it was almost 250 years old. All my intestines and stomach were releasing poisonous gases that would burn in the old days, so I nearly died. So, think of it like E. coli. What was happening in my body was bacterial abscesses sticking on the insides and everything. Now, I struggle with Lyme disease as an adult, but I don't reckon I really recovered. (Interviewee Tao)

Note: Lyme disease and MRSA were not connected conditions after an investigation by the Researcher.

Health challenges described by 30% of the survivors may be subjective as data was not obtained regarding whether a medical professional confirmed their diagnosis. However, a further 30% of the cohort stated that they did receive a formal diagnosis. None of the accounts has proven to associate child abuse with SPA directly. The Researcher compared the results from these studies with the previously compiled research. The Researcher discovered that the survivors and 1 MHP had described 28 previously unreported health conditions. The data included one count of leukaemia (blood cancer) and one mention of adolescent cancer reported by the MHP. Please refer to Volume Two, which includes the data and health information of the participants from the MHP study.

Among these conditions, one matched with a health challenge identified in the previous research conducted by (Felitti et al., 1998), which was asthma. Another condition mentioned by a survivor was prediabetes, which closely resembles diabetes (Kleinsorge & Covitz, 2012).

Importance of the Anomalous Health Data

In these studies, the Researcher has collected and incorporated anomalous data, some of which touches upon medical aspects, despite not being directly trained in the medical field. This decision stems from the unique perspective offered by survivors who shared their medical conditions during the interviews. As this thesis adopts a social constructionist lens, the Researcher aimed to investigate the intricate ways in which individuals construct their realities through communication and interaction within societal contexts.

Please note that the anomalous data collected during the PhD, albeit omitted due to word constraints, has now been reintegrated post-PhD completion as new content within this book. Additionally, the original PhD is recommenced in Key Theme Five. Furthermore, the Researcher has included the anomalous health data because she considered it her ethical obligation to report the information as the data may affect many child and adult survivors' lives.

Social constructionism guided the Researcher's choice to integrate anomalous data, encompassing survivors' perceptions of their medical conditions arising from SPA experiences. This decision stemmed from a desire to comprehend how these perceptions were shaped by personal and societal influences and how they were interwoven with the survivors and one MHP's collective interpretation of the world. The inclusion of this data aims to illuminate the complex relationship between individual narratives and the broader societal construction of reality. Additionally, adding this data acknowledges the social nature of human beings and encourages individuals to express their own narratives (Galbin, 2014). Doing so unravels the complexity and interconnectedness of various dimensions, including our personalised medical perspectives, that we often apply to ourselves and our surroundings to better understand who we are (Galbin, 2014).

The epistemological foundation of these studies is rooted in the assumptions of social constructionism. According to scholars like Berger and Luckmann (1991), socialisation occurs through communication and language with significant others who mediate the objective realities within society, giving them meaning and transmitting them to individuals. The individual then internalises this constructed reality. In this context, engaging in ongoing conversations becomes vital to sustaining, modifying, and reconstructing one's subjective reality (Andrews, 2012).

By incorporating medical data that emerged from survivors' narratives, the Researchers' intention is not to diagnose or analyse medical conditions but to acknowledge the perspectives and roles that these conditions played in shaping the survivors' experiences. During the interviews, the survivors often sought to find meaning in their experiences, and their medical conditions became intertwined with their stories. This epistemological stance aligns with the social constructionist approach, as it emphasises the importance of shared narratives and recognises that even medical aspects are socially mediated and interwoven with broader societal dynamics.

The data mentioned previously refers to the significant autoimmune diseases and potential links to cancers discovered in these studies from the anomalous data collected from the two cohorts, as described under 'Physical Health Manifestations' in the following pages. Additionally, the Researcher decided it is essential to include due to originality and contribution to knowledge as the majority of this data has not been collected before.

Furthermore, reporting this information may contribute significantly to the existing knowledge on potential links between SPA, autoimmune diseases, and cancer, which may currently affect an unknown number of SPA child and adult survivors. This previously uncaptured data also adds significant value to medical and mental health research. With so many people affected by PA and SPA worldwide, the information becomes crucial for preventing the further deterioration of their health conditions. By including these discoveries in the thesis, medical professionals can gain awareness of potential risks, enable early detection, and enact referral and intervention strategies to mitigate the influence of these conditions on patients' lives. Also, the reported cancer cases from the MHP and adolescents described in these studies highlight the urgent need for more research on this issue. Integrating this vital information into the thesis serves an ethical purpose, as it fulfils the responsibility of disseminating important research findings that may have profound implications for public health and patient care.

Furthermore, the thorough peer review process associated with a thesis ensures the credibility and validity of the research, ultimately contributing to the advancement of scientific knowledge that may have significant public health implications. The Researcher also has a moral obligation to disseminate important clinical findings that may impact the health and well-being of individuals. By reporting these findings, the research contributes to the advancement of scientific knowledge and allows MHPs and medical professionals to make informed decisions when providing care to patients with a history of PA and SPA.

Physical Health Manifestations

Key Theme Four explores the association between autoimmune diseases, common health conditions and cancer as reported by participants in both cohorts within these studies. For example, data reported on conditions mentioned in these studies include high cholesterol, cancer, leukaemia, adrenal fatigue, migraines, prediabetes, ulcerative colitis, irritable bowel syndrome (IBS), low zinc levels and more. The Researcher drew the associations from these studies' data and current peer-reviewed medical research findings. The findings suggest that survivors with many of the conditions described by the participants are also precursors to autoimmune diseases or are already autoimmune diseases.

Additionally, these studies indicate potential associations between the reported conditions, autoimmune diseases and cancer as reported in the current medical journals investigated by the Researcher. By reporting these findings, the associations can be used as a stepping stone for further research to enable healthcare professionals to diagnose and effectively manage symptoms potentially linked to SPA in child and adult clients and the MHPs who work with them. The MHPs are included because their data reports on the serious effect of working in the SPA field on their health as described in the upcoming section 'Occupational Cancer'.

Caveat Regarding Health Study

Important note: In discussing the newly introduced data in these studies, it is important to acknowledge certain caveats. Firstly, the Researcher reports that the presented information represents the perspectives of the survivors and one MHP from these studies. Additionally, the Researcher has investigated potential links to autoimmune disease and cancer from other peer-reviewed studies and compared the data to these studies. It is crucial to recognise that data from these studies may not have reached the level of support typically expected in rigorous research. However, it serves as a valuable starting point for future investigations to build upon.

By acknowledging the preliminary nature of this data, researchers can emphasise the need for further exploration and validation. It is worth noting that without capturing this early-level data on medical issues for survivors and MHPs, it could be a significant amount of time before another researcher emerges with similar findings. Therefore, despite the limitations and lack of prior capture, this data is a crucial starting place, offering a foundation for subsequent research endeavours. The scientific community needs to recognise the significance of this initial exploration and use it as motivation to advance the understanding and care for this population.

The following Table Five compiles reported anomalous physical conditions observed in these studies, along with related comparable research from current medical journals. It includes links to various survivor conditions, with a special category for autoimmune diseases and cancer.

The data highlights potential connections, but further research is needed to establish conclusive links between these conditions.

TABLE FIVE

Previous and Current Health Conditions of Six Survivors and 1 MHP

Reported Physical Conditions	Previously Collated Research (Felitti et al., 1998) (Perry, 2003), Downey et al., (2017).	Data from this Research Study (2022).	Survivor conditions & auto immune disease links.	Survivor conditions & autoimmune disease links to cancer.
Adrenal fatigue	-	✓	✓	-
Asthma	✓	✓	✓	✓
Blown discs in the spine	-	✓	✓	-
Brain damage (beatings from stepsister)	-	✓	-	-
Bulimia Nervosa	-	✓	✓	✓
Cancer-lung as an adolescent	-	✓	✓	✓
Cancer-nonspecific x 5 (reported by previous research) Leukaemia (blood cancer) x 1 (not reported by prev research) Data from MHP re colleagues) Total 6	✓ -	✓ ✓	✓	✓
Cancer in an adolescent client (reported by MHP) x 1	-	✓	✓	✓
Celiac Disease	-	✓	✓	✓
Chronic Fatigue	-	✓	✓	✓
Chronic Inflammation	-	✓	✓	✓
Chronic obstructive pulmonary disease (COPD)	✓	-	✓	✓
Colitis (Ulcerative)	-	✓	✓	✓
Diabetes	✓	-	✓	✓
Epigenetic changes	✓	-	✓	✓

Reported Physical Conditions	Previously Collated Research (Felitti et al., 1998) (Perry, 2003), Downey et al., (2017).	Data from this Research Study (2022).	Survivor conditions & auto immune disease links.	Survivor conditions & autoimmune disease links to cancer.
Fibromyalgia in the back, forearms and hips	-	✓	✓	✓
Hashimoto's Disease	-	✓	✓	✓
Heart disease	✓	-	✓	✓
High cholesterol	-	✓	✓	✓
Irritable Bowel Syndrome (IBS)	-	✓	✓	✓
Inflammation (unknown origin)	-	✓	✓	✓
Ischemic Heart Disease	✓	-	✓	✓
Liver Disease	✓	-	✓	✓
Low in zinc	-	✓	✓	✓
Lung Disease-Chronic	✓	-	✓	✓
Lyme Disease	-	✓	✓	✓
Migraines	-	✓	✓	-
MRSA (Methicillin-resistant Staphylococcus aureus)	-	✓	✓	✓
Obesity (post-study data not included)	-	✓	✓	✓
Petechiae (hemorrhage into the dermis)	-	✓	✓	✓
Poor self-related health- non-specific	✓	-	✓	✓
Post-Natal Depression (PND)	-	✓	✓	-
Pre-diabetes	-	✓	✓	✓
Post-traumatic stress disorder (PTSD) & Complex post-traumatic stress disorder (CPTSD)	-	✓	✓	✓
Pyroptosis	-	✓	✓	✓
Rheumatoid Arthritis	-	✓	✓	✓

Reported Physical Conditions	Previously Collated Research (Felitti et al., 1998) (Perry, 2003), Downey et al., (2017).	Data from this Research Study (2022).	Survivor conditions & auto immune disease links.	Survivor conditions & autoimmune disease links to cancer.
Stroke	✓	-	✓	✓
Sexually Transmitted Diseases	✓	-	✓	✓
Skeletal Fractures	✓	-	✓	✓
Thyroid Problem-Nonspecific	-	✓	✓	✓

Please note: Due to the restructuring necessitated by removing chapters from Volume One into Volume Two, some sequencing of the 'Tables' has been disrupted, resulting in an irregular flow. Please refer to Volume Two, 'Mental Health Practitioners', for the missing Tables as required.

In these studies, the data marked with red ticks correspond to the survivor cohort. These red ticks indicate a connection in the current medical research between the survivors' conditions and potentially auto-immune diseases. Furthermore, the red ticks extend to include current medical information on autoimmune diseases and cancers that survivors may be vulnerable to.

On the other hand, the data marked with green ticks represent health-related data collected from a single MHP participant in these studies. Notably, this participant's data stands out as the only instance showing anomalies related to autoimmune diseases or cancer links within the cohort of MHPs. The MHP's data has been combined with the data from these study's adult survivors' health conditions to provide a comprehensive overview.

Furthermore, the ticks in black are health data from previous child abuse studies. When the Researcher discovered further potential links to autoimmune diseases and cancers from these studies' data in the medical literature, which also built on the previously reported related parallel trauma research, namely 'adults who had experienced abusive child-hoods', these were combined and allocated yellow ticks.

The purpose of including the related previous medical literature was for the Researcher to conduct a comparative analysis, which led to the discovery of relevant medical connections between the survivors' known conditions, autoimmune diseases and cancers that may relate to survivors of SPA. The findings of these studies will be documented and shared with survivors, MHPs and medical professionals as potential conditions that may warrant careful monitoring. The subsequent section further elucidates the links between these conditions and autoimmune diseases and cancer:

Autoimmune Disease and Links to Cancer– A New Finding

A new research finding emerged while the Researcher investigated the survivors' and MHPs reported medical and health conditions data. Firstly, the Researcher noticed that within these studies' data, the 28 new health conditions reported differed from the previous data describing thirteen health challenges survivors might develop (Downey et al., 2017; Felitti et al., 1998; Perry, 2003). For example, celiac disease, Hashimoto's thyroiditis, Lyme disease, and colitis mentioned by study participants all fall within the autoimmune category (Global Autoimmune Institute, 2023).

Of note, the study by Felitti et al. (1998) was based on the relationship between health risk behaviour and disease in adults who had experienced abusive childhoods. This large study examined abuse and its connection to the extent of exposure to childhood emotional, physical, or sexual abuse, as well as household dysfunction during childhood. This study drew samples from a questionnaire on adverse childhood experiences from 13,494 adults who had undergone a standardised medical evaluation at a large health maintenance organisation (Felitti et al., 1998). The response rate was substantial, with 9,508 individuals (70.5% of the sample) participating in the study (Felitti et al., 1998). Their study did not mention PA or SPA, but it was chosen as a related parallel study to draw upon.

Due to this study being performed in 1998, the Researcher searched for an up-to-date study to compare the results further. The Researcher came across a study that replicated Felitti et al.'s (1998) study and reported that "chronic obstructive pulmonary disease" had been added to the original study findings (Downey et al., 2017, p. 557). Chronic obstructive pulmonary disease (COPD) is America's third leading cause of death (Downey et al., 2017).

Secondly, the Researcher discovered that, concerningly, 24 conditions described by six survivors in these studies were identified as autoimmune diseases or had links associated with autoimmune diseases. Thirdly, the Researcher discovered that 22 of these autoimmune conditions were reported as having the potential to escalate to cancer (Sakowska et al., 2022), as highlighted in red in Table Five. Additionally, the figure of 22 potential links did not include the seven confirmed cancer conditions collected from 1 MHP's data, as this figure is speculative. However, when the Researcher added all of the figures from the previous research and these studies, adult survivors and MHPs might be susceptible to 39 autoimmune diseases and 35 different types of cancer.

From this information, the Researcher then started investigating and including autoimmune diseases and links to cancer pertaining to these studies. Please note that the provided information is based on the data from these studies and three previous research reports and may not be an exhaustive list of all possible associations between autoimmune diseases and cancer among survivors and their MHPs.

Autoimmune disorders occur when an individual's immune system mistakenly targets and attacks their own body (Victorian State Government. Department of Health, 2021). These disorders encompass approximately 80 different conditions, varying in severity from mild to unbearable, depending on the specific body system affected and the extent of the immune response (Victorian State Government. Department of Health, 2021). The following survivor conditions drawn from these studies are listed for the reader and MHPs, and medical professionals to understand the links to associated diseases survivors may face, counteracting medical CITs further.

The inclusion of autoimmune disease and cancer in this thesis as a CIT for MHPs and medical professionals to be aware of was validated by recent research suggesting that autoimmune diseases develop due to the immune system's response against its antigens, leading to cancer arising when the immune systems fail to recognise malignant cells (Sakowska et al., 2022). This reference prompted the Researcher to look for links between autoimmune disease and cancer. Previously, autoimmunity and cancer have traditionally been viewed as distinct research areas with limited overlap (Sakowska et al., 2022). However, recent advancements in understanding immune checkpoints and the introduction of anti-cancer medications that target pathways such as PD-1 (programmed cell death receptor 1) and CTLA-4 (cytotoxic T lymphocyte antigen 4) have demonstrated the immense value of studying autoimmune diseases in the development of innovative anti-cancer therapies (Sakowska et al., 2022). The relationship between autoimmunity and cancer is complicated and has been described as "two sides of the same coin" (Sakowska et al., 2022, p. 1).

Survivor Autoimmune Conditions and Cancer Links

A recent study reports that individuals suffering from autoimmune disorders consistently exhibit a heightened susceptibility to cancer, which can arise from either an imbalance in their immune system or as an unintended consequence of medical interventions (Losada-Garcia et al., 2022). The correlation between the immune system and cancer is underscored by epidemiological evidence pertaining to cancer occurrence (Losada-Garcia et al., 2022). Subsequently, the Researcher discovered links between the majority of the conditions the survivors mentioned (reported in the following pages), autoimmune diseases and cancer. For example:

Celiac Disease

Celiac Disease is classified as an autoimmune disorder (Celiac Disease Foundation, 2023). Individuals with one autoimmune condition are more prone to developing additional autoimmune disorders (Celiac Disease Foundation, 2023). In the case of celiac disease, the risk of developing another autoimmune disorder increases with a later age of diagnosis (Celiac Disease Foundation, 2023).

Additionally, Celiac disease is also linked to other significant health conditions and certain types of cancer (Celiac Disease Foundation, 2023). These three types of cancer are non-Hodgkin's lymphoma, enteropathy-associated T-cell lymphoma (EATL), and adenocarcinoma of the small intestine (Beyond Celiac. Together for a Cure, 2023).

Hashimoto's Disease

Hashimoto's Disease is a disorder that can lead to an underactive thyroid, known as hypothyroidism (National Institute of Diabetes and Digestive and Kidney Diseases, 2021). In some rare cases, it may result in an overactive thyroid, referred to as hyperthyroidism. The thyroid gland, sited in the front of the neck and resembling the shape of a butterfly, is targeted by the immune system in individuals with Hashimoto's disease (National Institute of Diabetes and Digestive and Kidney Diseases, 2021). This immune response causes damage to the thyroid gland, impairing its ability to produce sufficient thyroid hormones. These hormones play a crucial role in regulating energy utilisation and impact the functioning of various organs, including the heart (National Institute of Diabetes and Digestive and Kidney Diseases, 2021).

Additionally, a comprehensive investigation by Hu et al. (2022) involving the analysis of 3,591 records was conducted to explore the potential connections between Hashimoto's thyroiditis and various types of cancer. After rigorous screening, 11 case-control studies and 12 cohort studies were deemed relevant for further analysis (Hu et al., 2022). The data analysis findings indicated that individuals with Hashimoto's thyroiditis face an elevated risk of developing certain types of cancer (Hu et al., 2022). Specifically, there was a notable association between Hashimoto's thyroiditis and breast cancer, urogenital cancer, digestive organs cancer, and hematologic cancer (Hu et al., 2022). These results suggest that survivors with Hashimoto's thyroiditis may require increased monitoring and preventive measures for these types of cancer.

Leukaemia

Leukaemia is a form of cancer that impacts both the blood and the bone marrow (Cancer Council, 2023). Leukaemia represents malignancies originating from the white blood cells and can be categorised in two primary ways: by the specific type of white blood cell affected, namely lymphoid or myeloid, and by the rate of disease progression and worsening (Cancer Council, 2023). Acute leukaemia manifests suddenly and exhibits rapid growth, whereas chronic leukaemia develops gradually, progressing slowly over months to years (Cancer Council, 2023). There are four specific types of leukaemia: acute lymphoblastic leukaemia (ALL), chronic lymphocytic leukaemia (CLL), acute myeloid leukaemia (AML), and chronic myeloid leukaemia (CML) (Cancer Council, 2023). Statistics suggest that over 5,200 individuals received a leukaemia diagnosis in 2022, with an average age of 65 (Cancer Council, 2023).

Chronic lymphocytic leukaemia (CLL) is associated with autoimmune disease (Diehl & Ketchum, 1998). The immune dysregulation observed in CLL is characterised by the presence of three autoimmune diseases: warm autoimmune haemolytic anemia (AIHA), idiopathic thrombocytopenia (ITP), and pure red cell aplasia (PRCA) (Diehl & Ketchum, 1998). The study by Diehl and Ketchum (1998) reports that approximately 11% of CLL patients in advanced stages experience AIHA. These autoimmune conditions primarily affect blood cells and are directly linked to the immune dysregulation observed in CLL (Diehl & Ketchum, 1998).

Lyme Disease

The Researcher found evidence linking Lyme disease to autoimmune disorders. This connection is supported by the presence of antibodies against self-tissue in the blood of individuals with Lyme disease, indicating the occurrence of autoimmunity. Furthermore, inflammation caused by Lyme disease can lead to damage in specific regions of the brain. Similar inflammation is observed in other neurological disorders, such as multiple sclerosis (MS) and Guillain-Barre syndrome (GBS), which are believed to be autoimmune diseases as well (MyaCare, 2023).

Additionally, there is a belief among scientists that bacterial infections, such as Lyme disease, have the potential to elevate an individual's risk of developing cancer by triggering inflammation within the body (Rees, 2021). Furthermore, these scientists estimated that infections and inflammation may contribute to approximately 25% of cancer cases (Rees, 2021). While the precise mechanisms behind this phenomenon remain uncertain, one hypothesis suggests that inflammation may induce DNA damage (Rees, 2021). Consequently, this damage can result in genetic mutations that can cause cancer (Rees, 2021).

Methicillin-resistant Staphylococcus aureus

Methicillin-resistant Staphylococcus aureus (MRSA) is a type of bacteria known as Staphylococcus aureus that is resistant to an antibiotic called methicillin and is the most prevalent form of staph infection (Australian Government Dept of Health and Aged Care, 2023). Infections caused by the difficult-to-treat MRSA bacteria can have a lasting detrimental impact on the lymphatic system, which plays a vital role in immune system functionality (McGreevey, 2018). These infections affect the skin or other soft tissues (McGreevey, 2018).

According to research conducted at the Mayo Clinic, prolonged exposure to minimal quantities of Staphylococcus aureus bacteria can potentially increase the risk of developing the chronic inflammatory disease known as lupus (Theimer, 2012). Staphylococcus aureus is a type of germ frequently present on the skin or within the nasal passages and can occasionally lead to infections (Theimer, 2012). In the Mayo Clinic study, mice were subjected to small amounts of a specific protein derived from staph, resulting in a lupus-like disease characterised by kidney complications and autoantibodies similar to those observed in the blood of individuals with lupus (Theimer, 2012).

Additionally, MRSA has been found to have significant implications for developing and progressing various types of cancers (Wei et al., 2022). Bidirectional effects of Staphylococcus bacteria have been observed in several cancer types, including skin, lung, bladder, colon, liver, lymphoma, breast, glioblastoma, and oral cancer (Wei et al., 2022). On the one hand, alterations in the staphylococcal flora within specific body tissues, such as the oral cavity, skin, or urinary system, have been associated with increased susceptibility to cancer or have been detected in cancer cases undergoing chemotherapy and/or radiotherapy (Wei et al., 2022). This data suggests a potential link between staphylococcal changes and cancer predisposition or treatment outcomes (Wei et al., 2022).

Petechiae

The Researcher discovered that petechiae is linked to Henoch-Schoenlein purpura (HSP) and are described as a rare inflammatory disease affecting small blood vessels (National Organisation for Rare Disorders, 2015). It is the most common form of childhood vasculitis (National Organisation for Rare Disorders, 2015), and HSP symptoms can occur suddenly (National Organisation for Rare Disorders, 2015). Inflammation can also occur in the joints, kidneys, digestive system, and central nervous system (National Organisation for Rare Disorders, 2015). The exact cause is not fully understood but is related to an abnormal immune system response (National Organisation for Rare Disorders, 2015).

Additionally, leukaemia and the associated rash are linked to petechiae (Moffitt Cancer Center, 2023). Under normal circumstances, platelets play a crucial role in blood clotting, preventing blood from escaping when a capillary breaks (Moffitt Cancer Center, 2023). However, platelet counts are reduced in cases of leukaemia which can disrupt the blood-clotting process (Moffitt Cancer Center, 2023).

Ulcerative Colitis

Ulcerative colitis (UC) falls within the category of inflammatory bowel diseases, encompassing similar conditions (Autoimmune Association, 2023). UC is classified as an autoimmune-related disorder characterised by inflammation and the formation of ulcers in the rectum and colon lining (Autoimmune Association, 2023).

Additionally, individuals diagnosed with UC face an elevated susceptibility to developing bowel cancer, which encompasses cancers affecting the colon, rectum, or bowel (NHS, 2022). This risk is particularly pronounced in cases where the condition is severe or involves a significant portion of the colon (NHS, 2022). Furthermore, the duration of UC is directly proportional to the magnitude of the associated risk (NHS, 2022).

Fibromyalgia

Fibromyalgia is described as an autoimmune disease (Kings College London, 2021). Recent research has shed new light on fibromyalgia symptoms, reporting that these symptoms originated in the brain rather than the immune system (Kings College London, 2021). Furthermore, this study suggests that many fibromyalgia symptoms are caused by antibodies that increase the sensitivity and activity of pain-sensing nerves throughout the body (Kings College London, 2021).

Additionally, exploring the relationship between cancer and fibromyalgia as comorbid conditions is an emerging field of research that still requires further investigation (Hanley, 2020). Several studies from

2001 have indicated a connection between the development of cancer subsequent to fibromyalgia or its symptoms and the occurrence of fibromyalgia following a cancer diagnosis, establishing a bidirectional association between the two conditions (Hanley, 2020).

Pyroptosis

Pyroptosis is an autoimmune disease characterised by the poor formation of cell membranes, cell rupture, and the release of pro-inflammatory cytokines such as IL-1β and IL-18 (You et al., 2022). Cytokines are small proteins secreted by cells that facilitate cell communication and interactions (Zhang & An, 2007).

Additionally, multiple scientific studies have provided evidence of a significant connection between pyroptosis and the progression and spread of numerous cancers (Wei et al., 2022). Various factors, including the activity of oncogenes, the immune microenvironment, and chronic inflammation, influence the development of tumours (Wei et al., 2022). Prolonged exposure to an inflammatory environment amplifies the likelihood of cancer development in cells and tissues (Wei et al., 2022). Additionally, pyroptosis has exerted anti-tumour effects in several cancer types, such as lung, gastric, breast, hepatocellular, and colorectal cancers (Wei et al., 2022).

Rheumatoid Arthritis

Rheumatoid arthritis (RA) is categorised as an autoimmune and inflammatory disease that occurs when the immune system mistakenly attacks healthy cells, leading to painful swelling and inflammation in affected body parts (Centers for Disease Control and Prevention, 2020).

Additionally, individuals with RA may face an altered risk profile when it comes to certain types of cancers (Worth, 2023). RA, a chronic autoimmune inflammatory ailment, manifests as joint pain and swelling (Worth, 2023). The likelihood of developing cancer can be influenced by various factors, such as the medications employed in RA treatment or the inflammation stemming from the disease (Bhandari et al., 2020). Although infrequent, RA patients exhibit an increased incidence of lymphoma, lung cancer, and skin cancer, while some other forms demonstrate reduced prevalence (Worth, 2023). Specifically, lymphomas, which are blood cancers, tend to be twice as likely to occur in individuals with RA compared to the general population (Gower, n.d). Non-Hodgkin's lymphoma and Hodgkin's lymphoma represent the primary classifications of lymphomas (Worth, 2023).

Chronic Fatigue

Chronic fatigue, known as myalgic encephalomyelitis, shares similarities with autoimmune illnesses and may be triggered by physical or emotional stress affecting the hypothalamic-pituitary-adrenal axis (HPA) (Centers for Disease Control and Prevention, 2018). In addition, fatigue can sometimes be linked to a different condition, such as anemia caused by cancer, although the exact cause of fatigue is often unknown (Rusin et al., 2022). Moreover, many individuals who have recovered from cancer continue to experience fatigue long after achieving remission, suggesting that these changes may persist as chronic symptoms in some instances (Rusin et al., 2022). These alterations may be transferred to offspring cells at a cellular level through inheritance or the maintenance of specific tissue micro-environments (Rusin et al., 2022).

Furthermore, while it is commonly recognised that chronic fatigue syndrome/myalgic encephalomyelitis (CFS/ME) and cancer are distinct diseases, there is a belief that they might share similar underlying causes in certain instances (Rusin et al., 2022). Cancer induces significant modifications in cellular metabolism, leading to proliferation and growth in oxygen-deprived conditions (Rusin et al., 2022). Based on previous studies, the researchers allege that CFS/ME also induces changes in cellular metabolism, potentially resulting in decreased energy production (Rusin et al., 2022). These researchers hypothesise that CFS/ME and cancer could be related conditions positioned along a spectrum of possible biological effects, with a general reduction in metabolism and growth in CFS/ME and enhanced anaerobic growth in cancer (Rusin et al., 2022).

Chronic Inflammation

Adding 'chronic inflammation of unknown origin' was important to include as a potential link, as abnormal inflammation has been linked to the pathogenesis of autoimmune diseases and various acute and chronic conditions (Storrs, 2022, p. 1). Additionally, inflammation is a natural response that aids in healing injured tissues (NIH National Cancer Institute, 2015). It initiates when damaged tissue releases certain chemicals, triggering the production of substances by white blood cells that promote cell division and tissue regrowth for repair (NIH National Cancer Institute, 2015). Additionally, the inflammatory process concludes once the injury is healed (NIH National Cancer Institute, 2015).

However, in cases of chronic inflammation, this process may commence without an actual injury and persist beyond its necessary duration (NIH National Cancer Institute, 2015). The reasons for persistent inflammation are unclear (NIH National Cancer Institute, 2015). Lingering infections can cause chronic inflammation, abnormal immune reactions towards healthy tissues, or conditions like obesity may also be contributing (NIH National Cancer Institute, 2015). Over time, chronic inflammation can damage DNA and increase the risk of developing cancer (NIH National Cancer Institute, 2015). For instance, individuals with chronic inflammatory bowel diseases like ulcerative colitis and Crohn's disease are more likely to develop colon cancer (NIH National Cancer Institute, 2015).

An interesting development occurred after the study was analysed when one of the survivors who had been included in the original data collection contacted the Researcher to add to her interview. The survivor revealed that she also struggles with obesity, a condition not originally captured during the interview and not included in the final conditions tally. However, while the information about obesity could not be included in the final conditions tally, it is still significant and relevant to these studies' findings. Although the survivor's obesity condition was not part of the original interview data, it is now acknowledged and mentioned here as an additional aspect to consider in understanding the complexities of SPA.

Bulimia Nervosa

Bulimia is a specific type of eating disorder and is identified as having a relationship with autoimmune diseases (Emamzadeh, 2019). The relationship between autoimmune conditions and eating disorders is bidirectional, indicating a potential shared underlying mechanism or risk factor (Emamzadeh, 2019). Research has shown that women diagnosed with any eating disorder have a 114% higher risk of developing an autoimmune illness within the following year (Emamzadeh, 2019). This risk decreases to 48% between the first and fourth year and 32% thereafter (Emamzadeh, 2019).

Additionally, bulimia among survivors increases the susceptibility to cancer by placing additional stress on the body, primarily through self-induced vomiting (Mauldin, 2023). This stress can weaken the body's defences against the development of cancerous cells (Mauldin, 2023). Squamous cell carcinoma is used when this condition is observed in the lining of the throat (Mauldin, 2023). The repetitive exposure of the throat to stomach acid in bulimia can cause small tears and cellular damage in the oesophageal mucosa (Mauldin, 2023). Over time, this damage can lead to complications such as gastroesophageal reflux disease and chronic physical harm (Mauldin, 2023). A study found a significant association between disordered eating behaviour and cancer, particularly oesophageal cancer (Mauldin, 2023). Individuals previously hospitalised with an eating disorder were found to have a six-fold increased risk of developing oesophageal cancer (Brewster et al., 2015).

Posttraumatic Stress Disorder

A research study discovered a correlation between PTSD (post-traumatic stress disorder) and later development in autoimmune diseases like rheumatoid arthritis, psoriasis, Crohn's disease, and celiac disease (Healthline Editorial Team, 2023). It is important to note that the Healthline study was observational, meaning it did not establish a direct cause-and-effect relationship between stress and autoimmune diseases that demonstrated an association (Healthline Editorial Team, 2023). The study's findings indicate that individuals who experience a stress-related disorder, such as PTSD, are more likely to develop autoimmune diseases (Healthline Editorial Team, 2023). However, further research is needed to establish a definitive causal connection between the two (Healthline Editorial Team, 2023).

Furthermore, PTSD can manifest in specific individuals following exposure to traumatic stress, according to a Swedish study that observed 106,000 people (Healthline Editorial Team, 2023). Alongside established psychological and behavioural symptoms, some individuals with PTSD exhibit increased levels of inflammatory markers, such as C-reactive protein, interleukin-6, and tumour necrosis factor-α (Katrinli et al., 2022). Additionally, PTSD frequently co-occurs with immune-related disorders such as cardiometabolic and autoimmune conditions (Katrinli et al., 2022). Several factors, including the cumulative burden of lifetime trauma, biological sex, genetic background, metabolic diseases, and gut microbiota, may contribute to inflammation in individuals with PTSD (Katrinli et al., 2022). Notably, inflammation can impact neural circuits and neurotransmitter signalling in brain regions associated with fear, anxiety, and the regulation of emotions (Katrinli et al., 2022).

Additionally, an analysis based on the Nurses' Health Study II data revealed a significant association between PTSD and an elevated risk of ovarian cancer, particularly among 44 premenopausal women (Levitan, 2019). The study utilised prospectively collected and self-reported information from 49,443 participants who were followed for 26 years (Levitan, 2019). Throughout a cumulative duration of 1,158,732 person-years, a total of 110 new cases of ovarian cancer were identified (Levitan, 2019).

Complex Post-Traumatic Stress Disorder

The Researcher conducted a Google search to explore the relationship between CPTSD, autoimmune diseases, and cancer. Previous research appeared to group PTSD and CPTSD together, despite their differing causes. For example, PTSD is typically associated with a one-time experience or single-incident trauma, as opposed to Complex Post-Traumatic Stress Disorder (CPTSD) which results from ongoing, inescapable, relational trauma (Brickel, n.d). Unlike PTSD, CPTSD involves being repeatedly hurt by another person, often resulting in betrayal and loss of safety (Brickel, n.d).

Furthermore, safe people, places, and things are essential for healthy brain development in childhood and adolescence (Brickel, n.d). Many adult survivors of complex trauma have experienced a loss of safety and lacked agency over themselves and their environment during critical periods of brain development (Brickel, n.d). This loss of agency has hindered their growth and denied them the opportunity to live fulfilling lives, resulting in a diminished sense of self-worth (Brickel, n.d). Even after escaping physical danger, these survivors live in constant hypervigilance and suffering (Brickel, n.d).

In addition to the mental and emotional effects, individuals with CPTSD who have experienced higher levels of childhood trauma are at increased risk for various health problems (Brickel, n.d). These include coronary heart disease (13%) and COPD (27%), as well as health risk behaviours such as smoking (33%) and heavy drinking (24%), according to the Adverse Childhood Experiences Study (Brickel, n.d). The severe impact of these effects often leads adult survivors to isolate themselves as a coping mechanism due to overwhelming feelings of unsafety

(Brickel, n.d). However, this isolation can result in despair and suicidality, perpetuating intergenerational cycles of trauma as their children may unintentionally adopt similar dangerous behaviours and coping strategies (Brickel, n.d). Based on this observation and the fact that the list of conditions for CPTSD is the same as for PTSD, the Researcher hypothesises that the risks of autoimmune diseases and cancer must be similar for both conditions.

Autoimmune Diseases Linked to Cancer from One Survivors Data

One survivor also described a cluster of medical conditions with potential links to autoimmune diseases. These were high cholesterol, adrenal fatigue, migraines, prediabetes, ulcerative colitis, and irritable bowel syndrome. Due to this list of conditions from one survivor, MHPs and treating doctors must remain open to the fact that survivors may present with more than one autoimmune disease, as previously reported in the celiac disease section (Celiac Disease Foundation, 2023).

HDL Cholesterol

Regarding cholesterol, a separate study was performed with a base cohort of 117,341 participants. The researchers discovered a significant correlation between low HDL cholesterol levels and heightened susceptibility to autoimmune disease among individuals in the general population (Madsen et al., 2019). However, it is crucial to acknowledge that the observational nature of their findings prevented them from establishing a definitive cause-and-effect relationship.

In addition, hypercholesterolemia could play a significant role in certain forms of cancer, such as breast and prostate cancer, as indicated by clinical investigations and animal studies (Ding et al., 2019). Nevertheless, due to inconsistent findings regarding the connection between hypercholesterolemia and cancer, the association between cholesterol and cancer may not be a straightforward two-way relationship (Ding et al., 2019). It is worth considering the possibility of an additional, conditional factor that could reverse the link between cholesterol and the advancement of cancer (Ding et al., 2019).

Adrenal Fatigue

Adrenal fatigue (also known as Addison's Disease) is an autoimmune disease that occurs when a person's immune system wrongly attacks healthy body tissues (Seladi-Schulman, 2022). No articles pertaining to any links between adrenal fatigue and cancer were found.

Migraines

Previous research reports a hypothesis suggesting that immunological changes, especially in migraine patients, may increase their vulnerability to developing immunological and autoimmune diseases (Biscetti et al., 2021). Conversely, specific pathogenic mechanisms associated with autoimmune disorders appear to contribute to the initiation of headaches in some cases (Biscetti et al., 2021). However, headaches were not reported in these studies.

Additionally, in a Danish study designed to examine the overall and site-specific cancer risk with individuals diagnosed with migraine, the researchers identified 72,826 patients who presented to the hospital with a first-time migraine diagnosis. Results concluded that their research could not support an association of cancer with migraine (Elser et al., 2021).

Obesity

As previously mentioned, under 'Chronic Inflammation', after the study data was collected, a survivor contacted the Researcher to add new information to her interview. She disclosed struggling with obesity, a condition not initially captured in the interview or included in the final tally of conditions. However, it remains noteworthy as a potential contributing factor to the complex CITs and conditions associated with SPA.

Strong epidemiological evidence supports a significant association between being overweight or obese and the risk of acquiring autoimmune diseases (Lerner et al., 2015; Jeremias & Matthias, 2015). From an immunological perspective, the association between being overweight or obese and the risk of developing autoimmune diseases can be explained by cellular and molecular mechanisms (Matarese, 2023). These mechanisms involve the overstimulation of T lymphocytes through nutrient- and energy-sensing pathways (Matarese, 2023). The immunometabolic state of an individual plays a central role in regulating immunological self-tolerance, which helps prevent autoimmunity by suppressing self-reactivity (Matarese, 2023). However, metabolic overload resulting from obesity can disrupt immunometabolism and potentially increase susceptibility to autoimmune diseases (Matarese, 2023).

Additionally, there is a clear association between being overweight or having obesity and an increased risk of developing 14 types of cancer which collectively account for 40% of all cancer diagnoses in the United States annually (Centers for Disease Control and Prevention, 2022). These cancers include "adenocarcinoma of the oesophagus, postmenopausal breast cancer, colon and rectal cancer, uterine cancer, gallbladder cancer, gastric cancer, kidney cancer, liver cancer, ovarian cancer, pancreatic cancer, thyroid cancer, meningioma, and multiple myeloma" (Centers for Disease Control and Prevention, 2022, p. 1)

Prediabetes

While Diabetes Type 1 or 2 were not listed in these studies, prediabetes was reported. An article on Type 1 and Type 2 diabetes explains that Type 1 diabetes is an autoimmune disease where the immune system attacks the insulin-producing cells of the pancreas, resulting in an insufficient insulin production and high blood sugar levels (Holland, 2022). On the other hand, Type 2 diabetes is characterised by insulin resistance and inadequate insulin production (Holland, 2022). While Type 2 diabetes has traditionally been viewed as a metabolic disorder, emerging research suggests it may also have autoimmune components (Holland, 2022). However, more evidence is needed to confirm this hypothesis and explore new treatment approaches (Holland, 2022). In summary, previous studies have revealed a significant link between prediabetes and autoimmune disease among survivors (Holland, 2022).

Additionally, data from 16 prospective cohort studies involving a total of 891,426 participants revealed that prediabetes is linked to a higher overall risk of cancer (RR 1.15; 95% CI 1.06, 1.23) (Huang et al., 2014). These findings remained consistent across various factors such as cancer type, age, duration of follow-up, and ethnicity (Huang et al., 2014). Different definitions of prediabetes did not significantly affect the risk of cancer (Huang et al., 2014). Regarding site-specific cancers, prediabetes was significantly associated with increased risks of stomach/colorectal, liver, pancreas, breast, and endometrial cancers (all $p<0.05$) (Huang et al., 2014). However, no significant association was found between prediabetes and bronchus/lung, prostate, ovary, kidney, or bladder cancer (Huang et al., 2014). Notably, the risks of specific cancers varied significantly ($p=0.01$), with liver, endometrial, and stomach/colorectal cancers having the highest risks (Huang et al., 2014).

Irritable Bowel Syndrome

Irritable Bowel Syndrome and recent research by pioneering gastroenterologist Dr Mark Pimentel, MD, reports that IBS in some of his patients could be an autoimmune disease (Kresser, 2023). Furthermore, irritable bowel syndrome and colon cancer symptoms can overlap with inflammatory bowel disease symptoms (City of Hope, 2021). Despite similar names, it is important to note that inflammatory bowel disease is distinct from irritable bowel syndrome and carries a significantly higher risk for colon cancer (City of Hope, 2021).

Colitis was mentioned earlier, so it is not discussed in this section.

Low in Zinc

Zinc deficiency is connected to a heightened vulnerability to infections and a greater likelihood of autoimmune diseases, as it disrupts tolerance mechanisms (Zahi et al., 2020). Patients with autoimmune diseases often exhibit low levels of zinc in their serum and plasma, suggesting that zinc may play a role either as a causative factor or as a contributor to the development and progression of these conditions (Zahi et al., 2020).

Additionally, having a low zinc concentration in the serum is an independent factor linked to an increased risk of cancer recurrence and an adverse prognosis (Nakanishi et al., 2022). Moreover, once zinc deficiency occurs, there is a higher likelihood of experiencing recurrent zinc deficiency (Nakanishi et al., 2022). Zinc deficiency can lead to various symptoms, such as hair loss, anemia, and taste disorders (Nakanishi et al., 2022). Lastly, the most prevalent causes of zinc deficiency are anemia and hypoalbuminemia (Nakanishi et al., 2022).

Previous Research- Autoimmune Diseases and Cancer

The Researcher examined potential links between previously compiled child trauma research by Felitti et al. (1998) and Perry (2021) and autoimmune diseases in current medical journals. The Researcher confirmed explicit connections between Felitti et al. (1998) and Perrys' (2021) childhood trauma condition list and autoimmune diseases in adults. However, it is important to note that the studies conducted by Felitti et al. (1998) and Perry (2021) did not specifically document any associations between child or adult trauma and autoimmune diseases. Consequently, the Researcher cross-matched Felitti et al. (1998) and

Perrys' (2021) conditions with current medical journals about autoimmune disease and concluded the following:

Chronic Obstructive Pulmonary Disease

Chronic Obstructive Pulmonary Disease (COPD) was reported by Downey et al. (2017) as an additional condition for adult survivors of abuse and their medical professionals to be aware of developing. A study conducted by Georgia State University and Vanderbilt University Medical Center analysed human genome information from Vanderbilt's DNA biobank and found that autoimmunity is involved in developing chronic obstructive pulmonary disease (COPD) (Georgia State University, 2018). COPD is a group of conditions that obstruct airflow and cause breathing difficulties (Georgia State University, 2018). It affects over 13 million people, and despite identifying specific genes associated with COPD through genome-wide association studies, the exact mechanisms behind the disease are not fully understood (Georgia State University, 2018).

People often equate COPD with heart disease, the leading cause of death in the United States, followed by chronic lower respiratory diseases like chronic obstructive pulmonary disease (COPD) (Cardio Vascular Institute Staff, 2017). These two conditions are often connected and share similar symptoms, such as shortness of breath (Cardio Vascular Institute Staff, 2017). Shortness of breath is commonly experienced by both COPD and Congestive Heart Failure (CHF) patients, especially during physical activity (Cardio Vascular Institute Staff, 2017). However, COPD includes chronic bronchitis and emphysema, causing irritation and damage to the airways and air sacs in the lungs (Cardio Vascular Institute Staff, 2017). This damage hinders the complete release of oxygen during exhalation, leading to shortness of breath (Cardio Vascular Institute Staff, 2017). While COPD and Congestive Heart Failure are distinct conditions with overlapping symptoms, there are also two other forms of heart failure (left-sided and right-sided) that may be influenced or worsened by the presence of COPD (Cardiovascular Institute Staff, 2017).

COPD is also linked to lung cancer (Parris et al., 2019). COPD and lung cancer are leading causes of mortality worldwide and share preventable risk factors like tobacco smoking and air pollution exposure (Parris et al., 2019). While only a small percentage of smokers (10-15%) develop COPD or lung cancer, the complex interchange of genetics, epigenetics, and environmental factors plays a crucial role in understanding these diseases (Parris et al., 2019). Although the exact mechanisms linking COPD to increased lung cancer incidence are not fully understood, recent studies provide compelling evidence of immune dysfunction, the lung microbiome, epigenetic regulation, and extracellular vesicles (EVs) in the development of both COPD and lung cancer (Parris et al., 2019).

Heart Disease

Heart disease was reported by both Felitti et al. (1998) and Perry (2021) and is known to be associated with autoimmune diseases (Conrad et al., 2022). This association implies that individuals with autoimmune diseases face a significantly higher risk of developing fatal and nonfatal cardiovascular diseases (Conrad et al., 2022).

Additionally, growing evidence indicates a heightened incidence of cancer among individuals with cardiovascular (CV) disease and heart failure (HF), with cancer often a leading cause of mortality in HF patients (de Boer et al., 2019). Recent research has demonstrated that circulating factors associated with HF contribute to tumour growth and development in animal models, establishing a causal link between the two conditions (de Boer et al., 2019). Multiple shared pathophysiological mechanisms connect HF and cancer, including inflammation, neuro-hormonal activation, oxidative stress, and impaired immune function (de Boer et al., 2019). Cancer frequently coexists as a comorbidity in HF patients, suggesting a pathophysiological association between the two diseases (de Boer et al., 2019).

Liver Disease

Liver disease was reported by Felitti et al. (1998) and is known to be associated with autoimmune liver disease (Beth Israel Deaconess Medical Center, 2022). Autoimmune liver diseases occur when the body's immune system mistakenly targets and attacks the liver, resulting in inflammation (Beth Israel Deaconess Medical Center, 2022). If not properly treated, this liver inflammation can progress and potentially develop into liver cirrhosis (Beth Israel Deaconess Medical Center, 2022). Cirrhosis increases the risk of developing liver cancer and can ultimately lead to liver failure (Beth Israel Deaconess Medical Center, 2022).

Lung Disease

Lung disease was also reported by Felitti et al. (1998) is linked to autoimmune diseases like sarcoidosis or rheumatoid arthritis (RA) (RA was reported in these studies), which increase the risk of developing interstitial lung disease (ILD) (American Lung Association, n.d). ILD encompasses various conditions that scar the lungs, making breathing difficult and hindering oxygen transfer to the bloodstream (American Lung Association, n.d). Unfortunately, ILD damage is often irreversible and worsens over time. Severe untreated cases can lead to serious life-threatening complications, including high blood pressure, heart or respiratory failure (American Lung Association, n.d).

Additionally, A study conducted in China involving 184 patients with interstitial lung disease (ILD) highlighted that ILD, particularly idiopathic pulmonary fibrosis (IPF) and connective tissue disease (CTD)-ILD, poses a risk factor for developing lung cancer (Xiaohong et al., 2021). Patients diagnosed with ILD-associated lung cancer (ILD-LC) generally have poor prognoses (Xiaohong et al., 2021). However, for those patients who can tolerate it, appropriate anti-tumour treatment can extend their survival time (Xiaohong et al., 2021).

In cases of mild ILD, targeted therapy and immunotherapy serve as viable alternative treatments for lung cancer patients (Xiaohong et al., 2021). Additionally, anti-angiogenic regimens have shown significant improvements in prognosis for ILD patients with advanced lung cancer (Xiaohong et al., 2021)

Poor Self Related Health

Poor self-related health (Felitti et al., 1998) is described as aiming to understand the social and biological mechanisms through which information from the human body is communicated to individual consciousness and how this information influences self-assessments of health (Jylha, 2009). However, Schmerling (2020) describes poor self-related health as 'stress' and suggests that stress could contribute to developing autoimmune diseases like lupus or rheumatoid arthritis (Shmerling, 2020). Additionally, the aforementioned study on stress has observed a higher occurrence of autoimmune diseases among individuals previously diagnosed with stress-related disorders (Shmerling, 2020).

Additionally, there may be an apparent connection between stress and cancer risk. However, it is important to note that the relationship between the two could be indirect (NIH National Cancer Institute, 2022). Chronic stress can lead individuals to adopt unhealthy behaviours such as smoking, overeating, reduced physical activity, or excessive alcohol consumption, all of which are known to be associated with an elevated risk of certain cancers (NIH National Cancer Institute, 2022).

Stroke

Extensive research has established a consistent link between stroke and autoimmune diseases (Felitti et al., 1998; Parikh et al., 2020). Individuals with autoimmune conditions are at a higher risk of stroke (Parikh et al., 2020). Additionally, around one-quarter to one-third of ischemic strokes are classified as embolic strokes of an undetermined source (ESUS) due to the lack of an established underlying mechanism (Navi et al., 2021). Furthermore, studies have also explored the association between stroke and cancer, suggesting a potential relationship, although further investigation is needed to understand the underlying factors and shared pathways involved (Navi et al., 2021).

Skeletal Fractures

Skeletal fractures (Felitti et al., 1998) can occur when a person has osteoporosis (Fletcher, 2023). While osteoporosis is not typically classified as an autoimmune condition by doctors, there is a growing understanding that the immune system and autoimmune processes may contribute to its development (Fletcher, 2023), which is why it was included in this section as a possible CIT to be aware of.

Additionally, bone density has emerged as a potential predictor of hormone-influenced cancers, including breast and endometrial cancers (NIH National Cancer Institute, n.d). In 1992, a clinical trial called FIT enrolled over 25,000 postmenopausal women to investigate the effects of alendronate on reducing osteoporosis fractures (NIH National Cancer Institute, n.d). The retrospective cohort study, known as BFIT, utilised data from the FIT trial to examine the relationship between hip bone mineral density and the risk of developing cancer (NIH National Cancer Institute, n.d). It also included a nested case-cohort study that explored the association between circulating sex steroid hormones and the risk of breast, endometrial, ovarian, and colorectal cancer (NIH National Cancer Institute, n.d). No results were reported for this study apart from the statement that ongoing endeavours are made to comprehend the connections between androgens and their metabolites and progesterone-related metabolites concerning the risk of breast cancer (NIH National Cancer Institute, n.d).

Sexually Transmitted Diseases

Sexually transmitted diseases (Centers for Disease Control and Prevention, 2020), also known as sexually transmitted infections (STIs), have been linked to the development of autoimmune diseases (Gupta, 2022). Several STIs, including Chlamydia, Hepatitis B, HSV-1 (herpes), and HIV (AIDS), have been associated with an increased risk of autoimmune disorders (Gupta, 2022).

Additionally, specific sexually transmitted pathogens have been identified as contributors to various types of cancer (NIH National Library of Medicine. National Center for Biotechnology Information, 1997). Specifically, certain strains of human papillomavirus (HPV) acquired through sexual activity are now recognised as the primary cause of cervical, vaginal, vulvar, anal, and penile cancers (NIH National Library of Medicine. National Center for Biotechnology Information, 1997). Hepatitis B virus, another sexually transmitted infection, is associated with hepatocellular carcinoma, a prevalent form of liver cancer (NIH National Library of Medicine. National Center for Biotechnology Information, 1997).

Additionally, specific cancers have been linked to other sexually transmitted pathogens (NIH National Library of Medicine. National Center for Biotechnology Information, 1997). Human T-cell lymphotropic virus type I (HTLV-I) is associated with adult T-cell leukaemia and lymphoma (NIH National Library of Medicine. National Center for Biotechnology Information, 1997). In contrast, human herpesvirus type 8 (HHV8) is linked to Kaposi's sarcoma, and Epstein-Barr virus (EBV) is implicated in lymphoma and nasopharyngeal carcinoma affecting the nasal cavity and pharynx (NIH National Library of Medicine. National Center for Biotechnology Information, 1997). Following on, the preceding collection of survivors, MHPs, and previously researched health conditions linked to autoimmune disease, cancer and associated conditions are presented in Table Six.

TABLE SIX

Health Condition Links to Autoimmune Disease, Cancer & Associated Conditions

AutoImmune	Associated Cancers	Associated Conditions
Bulimia Nervosa	Increased risk of developing cancer, particularly esophageal cancer. Squamous cell carcinoma.	Autoimmune disease. Eating disorders.
Celiac Disease	Enteropathy-associated T-cell lymphoma (EATL). Non-Hodgkin's lymphoma, Adenocarcinoma of the small intestine.	Autoimmune disease. Additional autoimmune disorders.
Chronic Fatigue	Fatigue can be linked to, and there may be shared underlying causes between, chronic fatigue syndrome/ myalgic encephalomyelitis (CFS/ME) and cancer.	Similarities with other autoimmune illnesses. Myalgic encephalomyelitis (ME). Anemia caused by cancer.
Chronic Inflammation	Colon cancer.	Autoimmune disease. Additional inflammatory diseases. Chronic inflammation. Chronic inflammatory bowel diseases link (e.g., ulcerative colitis, Crohn's disease).
Chronic Obstructive Pulmonary Disease (COPD)	Lung cancer.	Autoimmune disease. Shortness of breath. Chronic bronchitis. Emphysema. Type 1 diabetes. Rheumatoid arthritis Congestive Heart Failure. Left-sided and right-sided- Congestive Heart Failure.
Fibromyalgia	Fibromyalgia may be associated with cancer development or occur following a cancer diagnosis, establishing a biodirectional association.	Autoimmune disease.

AutoImmune	Associated Cancers	Associated Conditions
Hashimoto's Disease	Breast cancer. Urogenital cancer. Digestive organs cancer. Hematologic cancer.	Autoimmune disease. Hypothyroidism. Hashimoto's thyroiditis.
Heart Disease	Cancer frequently coexists as a comorbidity in heart failure patients, suggesting a pathophysiological association between the two diseases.	Individuals with autoimmune diseases face a higher risk of developing cardiovascular diseases. Links to autoimmune diseases. Links to fatal and nonfatal cardiovascular diseases.
High Cholesterol	Breast cancer. Prostate cancer (potential association, but not a straightforward relationship).	Autoimmune disease.
Irritable Bowel Syndrome	Overlapping symptoms with colon cancer, but irritable bowel syndrome itself is not associated with cancer.	Potential link to autoimmune disease. Inflammatory bowel disease
Liver Disease	Autoimmune liver diseases increase the risk of liver cancer.	Potential link to autoimmune disease. Liver cirrhosis.
Low Zinc	Zinc deficiency is associated with an increased risk of cancer recurrence and adverse prognosis.	Potential links to autoimmune disease. Hair loss. Anemia. Taste disorders. Hypoalbuminemia.
Leukaemia	Chronic lymphocytic leukaemia (CLL)	Warm autoimmune hemolytic anemia (AIHA). Idiopathic thrombocytopenia (ITP). Pure red cell aplasia (PRCA).
Lung Disease	Interstitial lung disease (ILD) poses a risk factor for developing lung cancer.	Links to autoimmune diseases sarcoidosis and rheumatoid arthritis. High blood pressure. Heart or respiratory failure.

AutoImmune	Associated Cancers	Associated Conditions
Lyme Disease	Infections and inflammation may contribute to approximately 25% of cancer cases.	Autoimmune disorder. Links to neurological disorders (such as multiple sclerosis and Guillain-Barre syndrome). Damage in specific regions of the brain. Bacterial infections. Links to genetic mutations that cause cancer.
Methicillin-resistant Staphylococcus aureus (MRSA)	Skin cancer, lung cancer, bladder cancer, colon cancer, liver cancer, lymphoma, breast cancer, glioblastoma, and oral cancer. Staphylococcal flora within body tissues, such as the oral cavity, skin, or urinary system, have been associated with increased susceptibility to cancer or have been detected in cancer cases undergoing chemotherapy and/or radiotherapy.	Staphylococcus infection. Lupus. Kidney complications. A potential link was reported between staphylococcal changes and cancer predisposition or treatment outcomes.
Headaches and Migraines	No significant association between migraines and cancer was found.	Links to immunological changes in migraine patients may increase vulnerability to developing immunological and autoimmune diseases. Specific pathogenic mechanisms associated with autoimmune disorders appear to contribute to the initiation of headaches.

AutoImmune	Associated Cancers	Associated Conditions
Obesity (captured from study participant-survivor after the study had concluded) *This condition is not included in the final tally.*	Adenocarcinoma of the oesophagus. Postmenopausal breast cancer. Colon cancer. Rectal cancer. Uterine cancer. Gallbladder cancer. Gastric cancer. Kidney cancer. Liver cancer. Ovarian cancer. Pancreatic cancer. Thyroid cancer. Meningioma. Multiple myeloma.	Links to autoimmune diseases. Type 1 diabetes (T1D). Multiple sclerosis (MS). Environmental and lifestyle factors contribute to an increased risk of multiple sclerosis (MS)= smoking, sun exposure, low levels of vitamin D, infection with the Epstein-Barr virus, and having a high body mass index (BMI).
Petechiae	Leukaemia.	Henoch-Schönlein purpura (HSP). Childhood vasculitis. Inflammation in joints, kidneys, digestive system, and the central nervous system.
Poor self-related health	Some connection between stress and cancer has been identified.	Stress-related disorders. Potential higher occurrence of autoimmune diseases- Smoking. Overeating. Reduced physical activity. Excessive alcohol consumption.
Post-traumatic stress disorder (PTSD Complex post-traumatic stress disorder (CPTSD)	Not directly linked, but PTSD and CPTSD may contribute to stress-related health issues that could potentially increase the risk of certain cancers, such as ovarian cancer in premenopausal women.	Mental health disorder. Observational links to autoimmune diseases- Rheumatoid arthritis Psoriasis. Crohn's disease. Celiac disease. Psychological and behavioural symptoms. Inflammatory markers-C-reactive protein, interleukin-6, and tumour necrosis factor-α. Cardiometabolic immune disorder. Impact on neural circuits and neurotransmitter signalling in brain regions associated with fear, anxiety, and the regulation of emotions.

AutoImmune	Associated Cancers	Associated Conditions
Prediabetes	Stomach/colorectal, liver, pancreas, breast, and endometrial cancers.	Autoimmune disease.
Pyroptosis	Lung cancer, gastric cancer, breast cancer, hepatocellular cancer, colorectal cancer.	Autoimmune disease.
Rheumatoid Arthritis (RA)	Increased incidence of lymphoma (blood cancers Non-Hodgkin's lymphoma and Hodgkin's lymphoma), lung cancer, and skin cancer.	Autoimmune and inflammatory disease. Joint pain and swelling.
Sexually Transmitted Diseases (STDs) Sexually Transmitted Infections (STIs)	Human Papillomavirus (HPV) is the primary cause of cervical, vaginal, vulvar, anal, and penile cancers. Hepatitis B is associated with hepatocellular carcinoma (liver cancer). Human T-cell lymphotropic virus type I (HTLV-I) is associated with adult T-cell leukaemia and lymphoma. Other STIs have been linked to specific types of cancer. Human herpes virus type 8 (HHV8) is linked to Kaposi's sarcoma, and Epstein-Barr virus (EBV) is implicated in lymphoma and nasopharyngeal carcinoma affecting the nasal cavity and pharynx.	STIs have been linked to the development of autoimmune diseases. Several STIs, including Chlamydia, Hepatitis B, HSV-1 (herpes), and HIV (AIDS), have been associated with an increased risk of autoimmune disorders.
Skeletal Fractures	Bone density may predict hormone-influenced cancers such as breast and endometrial cancers.	Osteoporosis. The immune system and autoimmune processes may contribute to the development of osteoporosis. Bone density. Ongoing research is being undertaken regarding links to breast, endometrial, ovarian, and colorectal cancer.

AutoImmune	Associated Cancers	Associated Conditions
Stroke	Potential links between stroke and cancer.	Autoimmune diseases increase the risk of- Stroke. Ischemic stroke. Embolic strokes of an undetermined source (ESUS).
Ulcerative Colitis	Bowel cancer (rectum or bowel). Increased risk of colon cancer.	Autoimmune disorder. Links to other inflammatory bowel diseases encompassing similar conditions.

Results From Table Six

From the data analysed in the summary Table Six, breast cancer was the most frequently mentioned condition. Following closely as the second most commonly mentioned were colon cancer, non-Hodgkin's lymphoma, lung cancer (noted in these studies), leukaemia (indicated in these studies) and skin cancer, each mentioned three times. Liver cancer was reported twice, while endometrial cancer, bowel cancer, urogenital cancer, and Hodgkin's lymphoma were mentioned twice. Glioblastoma, digestive organs cancer, hematologic cancer, prostate cancer, cervical cancer, vaginal cancer, vulvar cancer, anal cancer, penile cancer, hepatocellular carcinoma (liver cancer), and chronic lymphocytic leukaemia were mentioned once.

Additionally, nasopharyngeal carcinoma, chronic obstructive pulmonary disease (COPD), squamous cell carcinoma, Kaposi's sarcoma, and bone cancer were also reported once, highlighting a further 28 various cancer types and over 70 different combined health conditions and diseases that both cohorts may be susceptible to.

Furthermore, it is worth noting that the Researcher did not include the correlation between obesity and autoimmune diseases, as well as an additional 14 types of cancer (see Table Six) that emerged from post-study information on obesity in the final figures (Centers for Disease

Control and Prevention, 2022). These omissions were made to maintain the focus on the initially identified data from these studies and previous research. However, obesity is included as an added CIT for MHPs and medical professionals to be aware of, as mentioned.

The data in Table Six demonstrates that it is crucial to closely monitor the aforementioned health conditions among adult and child survivors of SPA and the MHPs who work in the SPA field. Monitoring is suggested due to the links between these conditions and autoimmune diseases, which can further impact the survivors' health and quality of life. Furthermore, these health conditions often have overlapping symptoms, shared underlying causes, or associations with other autoimmune disorders and chronic inflammatory diseases that may develop without proper monitoring procedures.

It is important to note that further research is ongoing to better understand the complex relationships and mechanisms underlying the links between autoimmune diseases and cancers. However, further efforts regarding these health conditions and SPA have not been mentioned. The evidence suggests that a comprehensive approach to monitoring and addressing these health conditions, alongside any mental health challenges relating to SPA, is necessary to ensure the long-term health and well-being of adult and child survivors of SPA and their MHPs.

Previous Findings Replicated in These Studies

The Researcher found that some of the survivors' diagnoses and symptoms from these studies were replicated within previous research reports regarding cancer. For example, the closest match was lung cancer (survivors' description), where at age 13, she received her diagnosis and had a lung removed. The second closest match was cancer-non-specific by Felitti et al. (1998), reported by an MHP regarding their colleagues and the adolescent client, as previously mentioned. No direct association between lung cancer and SPA was authenticated within the participant's answers. However, the MHP did believe that

SPA was a potential cause of her 14-year-old clients' cancer, stating, "There's severe alienation all over it" (ID withheld for confidentiality). As explained previously, further research would be prudent in validating this hypothesis.

Overall, these studies' findings (presented in the following sections) suggest a potential association between childhood trauma, SPA, and an elevated risk of developing a disease in adolescent and adult survivors and the MHPs working with them in the SPA field. While the data does not conclusively prove a direct link, the following results provide compelling evidence that warrants further investigation. Additional research is needed to thoroughly explore and validate this potential connection, considering confounding variables, sample size, and other possible influences on cancer development.

Child and Adult Physical Health Research in PA Studies

During these studies, the Researcher sought to investigate if other research had been conducted on physical health manifestations in child and adult survivors. Nothing specific was found in any PA textbooks or journal articles apart from the mention of somatic symptoms in children on the Australian web page titled "Alienated children (targeted)- The devastating impact on their mental health and life" in the for Eeny Meeny Miny Mo Foundation website (Eeny Meeny Miny Mo Foundation, n.d.). Physical health was mentioned once among the topics: "abandonment & trust issues, depression, anxiety, *somatic symptoms*, substance-related problems and suicide ideation and suicide" (Eeny Meeny Miny Mo Foundation, n.d.).

Continuing this quest, the Researcher explored studies focusing on physical health in children affected by PA and SPA. However, there was a lack of information on physical health and PA or SPA in peer-reviewed and grey literature, with only minimal mentions of somatic symptoms found. However, the Researcher did find a recent study with 1,212 participants from Europe in April 2023 validating the Researchers' brief investigation, reporting, "We have not been able to identify any studies from Nordic countries investigating the prevalence or health consequences of parental alienation" (Meland et al., 2023, p. 4).

These findings highlight the potential link between survivors' incidence of physical health symptoms and MHPs. These studies' results suggest that a comprehensive collaboration between MHPs, mental health professionals, medical personnel, and other relevant stakeholders begins to holistically address these physical health issues for the well-being of child and adult survivors and their MHPs.

Hypothesis by the Researcher

It is important to recognise the interconnectedness between physical and mental health, which appears limited in the context of SPA research. The focus on the psychological well-being of children in SPA cases may inadvertently lead to the neglect of their physical health symptoms, leading to adverse manifestations in adulthood. Physical symptoms could be attributed solely to stress or other non-specific causes, potentially delaying the recognition of underlying diseases or other physical health conditions. Within the following extracts, survivors share their convictions regarding the origin of physical symptoms, emphasising a strong belief in the role played by a life of exposure to SPA;

> I suffer with chronic fatigue. And that's because I've had so much lifelong stress from PA. And an important thing I think to bring up is that I had Pyro testing, and that's associated to stress. I've had fibromyalgia right down my forearms and down my back on my hips. That was a key indicator of, you know, some people say, oh, it's just a neurological, but it's like, you know, it's pain in your body. And living with that is not normal, where I had normalised it. (Interviewee Antje-Renee)

A male participant described how their symptoms had manifested mentally and somatically within his body, culminating in sleepless nights, inflammation, migraines, petechiae and CPTSD since childhood. This participant also commented that as an adult, the impact on his work life and study regarding his child abuse has been severe. The lifelong paradox he faced left him feeling faint and unable to act against his mother's abuse. This participant believed this had negatively impacted many parts of his life as an adult. The participant also explained that his poor physical and mental health severely impacted his dissertation, so he stopped just before finishing. The participant explained that he believed it was because he didn't trust anyone, and distrust was linked to his personal thought patterns. He shared this example of his thoughts;

> I saw the counsellor making me want to help my tormentor as they felt sorry for her. Even today, the false comments my mother made to me makes me faint, unable to act. All of this had a negative impact on my physical health. I had 90 per cent of my dissertation finished. I stopped because I was convinced that I was too bad and didn't deserve it. In my dissertation, I collected and examined more than 9000 subjects (hemodynamic, etc., under stress), but I can't finish it mentally or physically. Every day, I feel weak in my body, not worth living. I miss my father but can hardly see him, get mad at my mother, then at myself and so on. But I have two wonderful boys. I have to move on. (Interviewee Shane)

The curiosity surrounding a way to start to repair a relationship with one's inner child was highlighted by an observation from a survivor who mentioned that she had been wandering through a small book section at work and noticed a book about helping your inner child. She shared that she didn't pick it up but wondered what the book could be about because she couldn't read due to her childhood trauma of abduction and SPA and how it had physically affected her brain and her ability to focus;

> And I looked at this book, and I remember seeing a white silhouette of a child, and there was light behind it. And I remember looking at it, and I went walking, and I sat down, and I had my lunch. And I was thinking about my inner child. And I thought, what would that book be about? And I couldn't read because of what had happened to me. If I tried to read, I wouldn't remember what I was reading. So, it was really hard. My brain just couldn't focus. (Interviewee Antje-Renee)

Conclusion

In conclusion, this study highlights the significant yet underexplored relationship between psychological abuse, specifically in SPA, and its potential impact on physical health. Prior research has revealed a compelling link between childhood trauma and adverse health outcomes, focusing on potential cancer risks and other health challenges. The findings underscore the need for a comprehensive and interdisciplinary approach to comprehending the intricate interplay between psychological and physical well-being, particularly among survivors of SPA and MHPs working within this field.

The emergence of previously unreported health conditions among survivors and MHPs and the potential associations with cancer raise important questions that require thorough investigation. Collaborative efforts are essential to explore the underlying factors contributing to the MHPs observed health challenges. Further research must delve into potential environmental, occupational, and shared risk factors that could be influencing the increased incidence of cancer and other health conditions. Moreover, the connections highlighted between chronic stress, burnout, and physical health challenges emphasise the importance of a holistic approach, considering the complex interaction between psychological and physiological well-being.

KEY THEME FIVE

Survivor Insights, Resilience and Challenges

Adaptation From Trauma

The lived experience of SPA was different for all of the participants in the study. As many survivors have experienced overwhelming challenges growing up as children of SPA, they described methods of adaptation that included the development of personal resilience and insights, coping styles, and protective self-care factors. Figure Seven summarises the personal insights and challenges from survivors regarding their levels of resilience and how family members have helped. Survivors also described their loss of hope about SPA ever ending, negative thoughts about themselves and how the feeling of abandonment affects their lives.

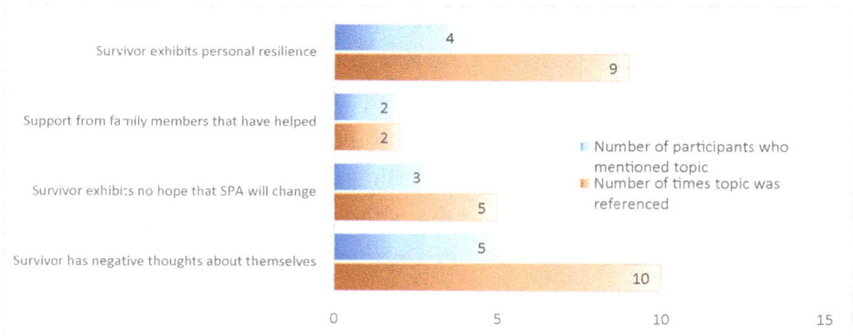

FIGURE SEVEN
Survivor Insights of Their Own Personal Resilience and Challenges

> There is definitely different levels of severity, and although there's still trauma, probably on every single level. At severe levels, we're most often cast aside or ignored. We're not broken. We might be broken temporarily, but we can work through this. And it takes effort on our part, and it takes knowledge and know-how from our MHPs. And together, we

> can heal faster. Because it's taken me over a decade to get to where I'm at. (Interviewee Aurora)

Others developed differently, such as comparing and watching other community members. For one survivor, the road to acceptance has been hard fought;

> Didn't matter who I met, they could have been from any walk of life, and I was less than they were. My needs were less important than theirs were. My voice wasn't as relevant as theirs was. It wouldn't matter. It wouldn't matter if they were dead drunk on the pavement and just spouting bullshit. For me, anybody, any human that I met, was better than me. Any human, anything they said was more right than anything I said. Yes. That was before therapy. But now it's – I've probably swung the other way because I guess my basic philosophy is that people are shit. But I guess I'll swing back to some sort of equilibrium, but I don't know, there's so much evidence to support that [laughter], it's ridiculous, and it just keeps going, it's just true. But yes, there are some good people, not me, but – yes, so that's the difference, I guess. Just people who just prod, who just provoke you, who just goad, and it's devastating. But now, I wouldn't respond the same way. I have a voice now, whereas before, I didn't, and I just froze, and it's triggering. (Interviewee Alan)

Health Literacy-Labelling Emotions and Experiences

This section collected and summarised the health literacy language obtained when the survivors spoke about healing stories. Under the heading of health literacy, 30 references from six adult survivor participants were recorded. Topics pertaining to the survivors' health included commentary on boundaries, identity, attachment theories, reconnection, reactive stage, reframing, gaslighting, psychological abuse, psychotherapy, active listening, empathy, regulating others, reregulating oneself, encroachment, and dysregulation. Also mentioned were enmeshment, talk therapy, overreacting, guilt language, attachment styles, fearful avoidant, cognitive, intergenerational trauma, unconditional positive regard, CPTSD, abduction, severe childhood trauma, and trauma-informed. Lastly, the ACE Study, being present, love bombing, diplomacy, generalised anxiety, and anxious preoccupied. Counterintuitive alienation, listening blocks, schemas, repressed positive memories, and repressed trauma were listed.

With many of these traits commonly associated with suicidal behaviours, it is significant to highlight SPA's effect on individuals. This list indicates a need to; increase the profile and supply of SPA health promotion programs within the general community, educate mental health professionals on the extensive issues of SPA, monitor the levels of resilience concerning psychological and physical manifestations and continue to develop health promotion programs to increase the awareness of living with child abuse trauma that may last a lifetime. Furthermore, the survivors' requests for more education by improving their mostly self-taught education and health literacy of the survivors and their families need to be heeded. There is a need for additional discussion and research on the impact of suicide and risks and protective factors within the adult survivor's world. This will help to encourage the development of policies and provide funding and access to specialise suicide prevention programs for survivors.

Summary

In conclusion, Chapter Five aimed to provide clinical insights into the experiences and perspectives of survivors of SPA. The findings illuminated the intricate social dynamics and the profound impact of child psychological abuse on these individuals. One significant theme that emerged was the negative experiences with MHPs reported by the participants. The lack of psychological safety in therapeutic settings and the limited understanding of SPA by MHPs hindered the survivors' ability to seek help and find effective support. This theme highlights the need for improved education and training for MHPs to understand better and address the unique challenges faced by survivors of SPA.

Additionally, the study revealed the survivors' perspectives on therapy outcomes and their comparisons between MHPs and their own experiences. The participants expressed a desire for more comprehensive education and training on SPA, both for MHPs and themselves. The cost of therapy and its accessibility through the Australian Medicare system were also identified as challenges, particularly for those with limited health literacy. The chapter also explored the mental health aspects of survivor experiences, uncovering various adverse psychological encounters.

The survivors also shared their struggles with identity, suicidality, phobias, and paranoia, highlighting the profound impact of SPA on their mental well-being. False allegations of CSA and the long-lasting effects of abduction during childhood were additional topics of discussion, emphasising the complexities of survivors' journeys towards healing and recovery. These studies also uncovered the survivors' perspectives on adaptation from trauma and the importance of health literacy in labelling emotions and experiences.

Summary of Research Discovery

Significant clinical themes emerged and identified potential novel diagnostic indicators. These findings offer crucial clinical implications, empowering MHPs to better understand and monitor the well-being of SPA survivors within a clinical context. For example, the Researcher reported the discovery of a "specific phobia-severe parental alienation, and abduction anxiety variant" (Price-Tobler, 2023), along with information regarding FDIOA and malingering by proxy.

In addition, the discovery of a high prevalence of cancer among the MHPs who work within the SPA field is also noteworthy. These findings serve as a reminder of the extensive toll that SPA can take on individuals' overall well-being. Recognising and addressing these physical health issues is essential to provide comprehensive support for survivors and MHPs through their treating professionals.

Drawing from the experiences shared by the survivor participants, who emphasised the significance of taking control of their emotional landscapes for healing and resilience, the upcoming Chapter Six shifts focus to the MHP cohort. This chapter explores the results obtained from MHPs involved in these studies, shedding light on their professional perspectives and contributions to further understanding clients needing support with SPA.

Please note: Due to the restructuring necessitated by removing chapters from the twin study PhD, the sequence of chapters and appendices has been disrupted, resulting in an irregular flow between Volume One and Volume Two. Consequently, some chapters may not appear sequentially, which may appear unusual to readers.

Chapter Seven

Study One Discussion and Conclusion-Adult Survivors of SPA

Firstly, readers should note that research regarding the effects of SPA on adults who experienced this phenomenon as children is a relatively new field. Consequently, much remains to be discovered about the impact of SPA on affected individuals. Nevertheless, these studies effectively addressed its initial Study One aim: to investigate the perspectives of survivors who seek treatment from MHPs. Specifically, these studies explored the survivors' opinions regarding the effectiveness of therapy, areas where therapy fell short, and recommendations for improving survivors' therapeutic relationships with MHPs.

The following chapter underscores a range of significant discoveries from the study. These encompass CITs and the deficiency of SPA knowledge among MHPs. Additionally, the chapter sheds light on survivors' substantial contributions to mental and physical well-being knowledge and explores the adoption of a contemporary perspective within the SPA field. It also delves into the lack of survivor recognition and offers a new, more positive lens through which the survivors would like to be viewed, followed by recommendations to enhance therapeutic practices. Survivor insights are elucidated on crucial topics, psychoeducation, ethical dilemmas, and mental health and identity challenges.

Moreover, this chapter acknowledges study limitations, including sample size and potential insider researcher bias, while suggesting future research avenues involving lived experience practitioner-researchers, evidence-based guidelines, and increased involvement in decision-making processes. In addition, this chapter presents higher-level arguments that have emerged from the data, such as the resourcefulness of survivors despite feeling underestimated in earlier research on PA. Furthermore, the study reports a misrepresentation of survivors through omission, indicating a lack of recognition of their valuable contributions to research, PA organisations, symposiums, and advocacy.

Findings of the Study

The present findings indicate that survivors who seek therapy from MHPs for their symptoms face considerable difficulties. To add to future research, these studies gathered and collated data on these reported psychological, physical, and social dimensions and CITs. CITs are a concept developed by the Researcher and are described as important tributaries of SPA abuse that add to the knowledge regarding what survivors have been exposed to. In addition, CITs are important SPA client presentations that MHPs need to be aware of to counteract disguised presentations (Gelinas, 1983).

MHPs Lacking SPA Knowledge

Survivors shared their perceptions of practitioners lacking knowledge regarding SPA. For example, they noticed that MHPs are uncertain about which modalities and therapies to apply when in session with the survivor and how and when to administer them. Interestingly, the data shows that the survivors consider their knowledge of SPA high due to self-education efforts. Hence, the survivors took it upon themselves to train their MHPs (not study participant MHPs as they are different) during therapy sessions to counteract this anomaly.

Many degrees among the survivor study participants raise an intriguing question, considering the existing negative narratives on children who experience SPA. Previous research has highlighted the impacts, including school-related issues, such as disruptive behaviour, social withdrawal (Clawar & Rivlin, 2014), truancy, and variations in academic performance (Haines et al., 2020). The research also indicates that some alienating parents prioritise their own needs over their children's educational requirements, leading to irregular school attendance (Haines et al., 2020).

Given these findings, it becomes perplexing to understand why the survivors participating in the study, who have experienced SPA, report high levels of university education, professional training, and over twenty degrees between them. This contrast between the educational background of the survivor participants and the adverse outcomes observed in children experiencing SPA challenges the current understanding and prompts further examination of the factors influencing educational attainment and resilience among survivors of SPA.

Significant Contributions to Mental and Physical Health by Survivors

The findings indicate that survivors can make valuable contributions to mental and physical health research and training. This finding is noteworthy because, despite the obstacles they have faced as survivors, they have demonstrated the ability to overcome them and become experts based on their own lived experiences. As a result, survivors can provide valuable input in future research, symposiums, advocacy, and organisations that focus on survivors, paving the way for a more contemporary approach to these issues.

These studies recommend that MHPs acknowledge the expertise and knowledge of SPA survivors and engage them in the therapeutic process as partners. MHPs should remain curious and incorporate the survivors' self-education on SPA and the social dimensions they have experienced when in session. In psychotherapy, the survivors are often considered the experts on themselves. This psychotherapeutic lens differs from other psychology professions where the MHP professes to be the expert on the client, allowing for little input from the survivor. The study also recommends that survivors should be engaged as partners to create a more collaborative therapeutic environment that fosters trust and empowerment while contributing to the field of research. Additionally, the study suggests that future research should explore how and why survivors with high levels of literacy and educational degrees went to such lengths to understand their SPA experiences during treatment so that other survivors can improve engagement in therapy.

Adoption of a Contemporary Lens in the SPA Field

According to Bill Gye, OAM and CEO of Community Mental Health, Australia, "traditional medical practices, such as psychiatry and clinical psychology, retain, to a considerable degree, outdated power structures that place medical professionals at the top of the hierarchy. At the same time, the patient and their families are relegated to the bottom" (B. Gye, personal communication, May 3rd, 2023).

Mr Gye also reports that "such a hierarchy undermines values like respect, involvement, and inclusion". On the positive side, this arrangement is gradually being modified in many Australian organisations, particularly in the community-managed sector. "This modification is being achieved by adopting a more contemporary lens combined with practices of recognition, support, and inclusion of lived experience participants" (B. Gye, personal communication, May 3rd, 2023).

The Researcher argues that Mr Gyes' viewpoints ought to be implemented in the field of SPA and proposes that a more equitable power distribution is necessary if the relationships between survivors and MHPs are to advance. Creating a culture that values the input of survivors and their families is crucial and empowering them to be active participants in decision-making processes can improve the quality of care and establish a more inclusive and supportive environment.

Lack of Survivor Recognition

These studies also report an undercurrent of 'lack of recognition' regarding the SPA survivors' experience within the PA community of professionals and the generalised mental health community. It is important to note that despite the valuable study insights provided by survivor study participants, the survivors reported knowing only one survivor they noticed speaking at conferences or participating in the larger PA organisations. The survivors also report that many of the self-named 'experts' in PA organisations and conferences do not have lived experience of SPA as a child that they are aware of, making them question some of the lenses through which the research data is analysed. For example, one of the MHP study participants listed an example of typical PA conference speakers as psychiatrists, researchers, clinical psychologists, and lawyers who litigate for the parents involved in high-conflict divorce.

The survivors report believing they hold the key to stopping SPA. However, one MHP study participant describes that the PA experts repeatedly monopolise the guest speaker's line-up and do not consider that they are talking about survivors who are watching. Survivors report that this leaves them feeling unseen, unrecognised, and undervalued. In addition, the limited inclusion of lived experience survivors from conferences and professional organisations raises concerns about the motto, 'nothing about us without us,' which is the motto shared by survivors who feel they are not given a larger, more supportive, valued platform to voice their experiences and insights. One survivor participant "Aurora" shares, "We are tired of being just study research participants". Thus, the study recommends that more than a token gesture be made regarding the inclusion of survivors in conferences, meetings, and other platforms, and this significant issue requires immediate attention and action. For example, the majority of the 'Schizophrenia Fellowship of NSW Ltd (trading as One Door Mental Health)' Board comprises lived experience consumers as part of their Constitution (One Door Mental Health, 2020).

A Contemporary Comparison

These studies suggest that professionals working with survivors in the field of SPA should adopt a contemporary approach and recognise the valuable contributions these survivors can make to the field. For example, in Australia, several forward-thinking organisations such as 'One Door,' Flourish, Mind, NEAMI, Wellways, RUOK, Suicide Prevention Australia, and Postvention Australia now appreciate and incorporate people with personal experiences of mental illness, survivors of complex trauma and their families, staff, health professionals and advisors. In addition, lived-experience consumers and carers now hold positions on these committees and Boards. Furthermore, they share their perspectives and stories at symposiums and participate in research, training, and psychoeducation programs.

Mr Bill Gye emphasises the importance of incorporating people with lived and learned experience within the governance and management of organisations (B. Gye, personal communication, May 3rd, 2023). Mr Gyes' view is that having at least two or three people with lived experience (as consumers or carers) in all organisational meetings is necessary to address the historical imbalance and can help ameliorate the common practice of having just one token consumer. In addition, progressive organisations increasingly recognise the value of having people on their teams who combine their personal experience as consumers (or carers) with studied knowledge of the topic at hand ("lived and learned experience"). Furthermore, Mr Gye states that by combining personal experience and academic knowledge, organisations can create a potent force for driving progress to produce much better outcomes for all people who have experienced mental or physical health challenges (B. Gye, personal communication, May 3rd, 2023).

The Researcher argues that professionals in the SPA field should adopt an inclusive and contemporary view of survivors, recognising their contributions. Incorporating individuals with lived and learned experience into the governance and management of organisations can redress historical imbalances and improve outcomes in psychology. Therefore, these studies recommend that professionals take proactive measures to include survivors and their families in advancing the PA and SPA field.

Recommendations for Improved Therapeutic Practice

Based on these studies' findings, improving professional practice among MHPs when working with survivors is imperative. For example, all mental health professionals working with survivors should be familiar with and skilled in the many types of childhood trauma and CITs that an adult survivor may have experienced, such as manipulative strategies that have brainwashed them as children (Baker, 2007). Knowing that ten survivors report having an unrecognised disguised presentation, it is likely that most community professionals will come across survivors either knowingly or unknowingly in their careers. In addition, professional development regarding SPA and CITs will equip mental health professionals who typically only focus on diagnosable disorders and how to treat them. Herman (1992a; 1992b) noted that the diagnostic criteria for diagnosable disorders are not designed for or met by survivors of repeated trauma experienced during the child development stage.

Brainwashing

According to earlier research, survivors have reported being subjected to "emotional manipulation strategies," such as withdrawing love, creating dependency, and forming loyalty binds by their AP (Baker, 2007, p. 12). Additionally, survivors describe the use of brainwashing techniques by the AP in the form of repetitive negative statements about the TP and black-and-white thinking (Baker, 2007, p. 32). Early research characterises this as "the cult of parenthood" and identifies the brainwashing or programming of children as a critical element of parental alienation (Baker, 2007, pp. 32, 84).

Within these studies' results, the survivor participants spoke about knowing they had been brainwashed but did not know how to reverse the damage. Many survivors' data included narratives describing the primary manipulation brainwashing techniques used to invoke fear, persuade, control, and manipulate children (Baker, 2007, p. 84). According to psychiatrist Dr Robert Jay Lifton (1969), the five brainwashing techniques align with thought reform techniques (Baker, 2007). These techniques create psychological stimuli in the environment that impact the individual's emotions and align with the brainwashing methods distinguished by Clawar and Rivlan (1991). According to Baker (2007), programming relates to the message's content, while brainwashing pertains to the techniques used to convey the message.

This Researcher reports that the survivor participants also had these brainwashing narratives within their interview data, and many still live with the effects of the manipulative techniques used by their AP. These are interesting results as previous research has been limited regarding whether survivors still feel the effects of brainwashing from their childhoods and if they ever find a way to recover from the techniques they were exposed to as children.

Psychological Safety

In this section, survivors identified their perceptions and risks of revealing historical and current trauma and abuse stories to MHPs. These were described as the MHPs appearing to be running the session, seeming shocked, looking uncomfortable, and becoming vicariously traumatised themselves. Also reported were confusing emotions where MHPs maintained a blank therapeutic attitude and showed little empathy or compassion.

Furthermore, survivors reported that MHPs were too treatment-focused, had limited time and flexibility, recommended inappropriate referrals and strategies, and left the survivor without treatment while taking their money and suggesting they return. Finally, survivors interpreted the MHPs' behaviour as uncomfortable, and that the survivor was 'too hard and complex' to deal with. The survivors also noted that some MHPs would change the survivors' topics during the session to something more palatable. Consequently, some survivors shut down and stopped trusting the practitioners.

Survivors also reported being worried about the MHP's reactions and whether their story was too much for the therapist to hear when they spoke about their trauma. As a result, the survivors reported having to 'regulate' the therapist and only share small parts of the trauma once they had gathered that the MHP could handle their stories. Consequently, many survivors did not feel psychologically safe due to the MHP's biases and characteristics stemming from sociocultural myths, standards and personal expectations revealed within the session (Alaggia, 2010; Sorsoli et al., 2008).

Survivor perspectives were also drawn from the MHP's ability to listen and be empathetic, demonstrating the MHP's level of discomfort when hearing their material. The study reports that the MHPs being self-aware and honest was particularly important to the survivors and that practitioners must be mindful if they are conveying discomfort as this may lead the survivor to feel shame and judgement.

Negative Reflections Regarding Sessions with MHPs

In the eleven interviews, the survivor participants shared forty-eight negative experiences related to their interactions with MHPS. The reflections indicated that some survivors may have had challenging experiences receiving support for SPA-related trauma. These studies recommend that MHPs know the risks that survivors perceive when disclosing trauma stories. MHPs must be self-aware of their reactions and biases to create a safe and supportive environment for the survivor. MHPs must listen with empathy and unconditional positive regard (Rosenberg, 2015) to avoid a solely treatment-focused approach that may not be appropriate for the survivor's unique needs. Additionally, MHPs must be flexible with their time and treatment options and willing to make appropriate referrals with input from the survivor. Finally, MHPs need to ensure that survivors feel safe and validated while acknowledging the complexity and severity of the trauma and not dismissing it as 'too hard' to deal with.

The survivor participants cited an absence of hope due to a lack of education about SPA for MHPs and feeling they would never find anyone who understands their child abuse trauma. This data indicated a need for self-agency skills to be taught by MHPs to survivors and more education to be undertaken if the practitioner is to work with survivors and protect their psychological safety. Loss of hope was also attributed to a lack of recognition for the survivors. This lack of recognition was ascribed to the feeling that the larger, more research-based PA organisations are leaving them out and do not recognise their value and experience.

Helpful Ideas, Topics, and Psychoeducation as Recommended by Adult Survivors

Within Key Theme Two, eight survivors listed forty-one references to the question, "What types of therapy was tried or suggested by the practitioner?" The therapies included medical model therapies, cognitive behaviour therapy, eye movement desensitisation, and reintegration therapy. Also mentioned were holistic approaches, such as massage therapy, nature therapy, and reiki.

In addition to the treatments they received, survivors shared sixty-nine different ideas, topics, and psychoeducation subjects that they found helpful in therapy. Many were holistic and educational, including sports, physical bodywork, art, journaling, and psychoeducation. For instance, survivors suggested seeking domestic violence support, overcoming brainwashing and gaslighting, learning to regulate their emotions, practising yoga Nidra, using music therapy, and implementing mental health strategies. This list indicates that the MHPs and the survivors believe that a combination of medical and holistic approaches may be most effective in treating SPA. The most effective way to test this hypothesis would be in clinical trials with survivors and MHPs working together. The survivors' perspectives on the therapies applied by MHPs to treat SPA highlight the need for a combination of evidence-based and holistic treatment models to guide practitioners. For an integrated approach to fruition, the MHPs and survivors must find various successful medical and holistic methods together. In addition, referrals and collaboration with other specialist professionals will need to be actively sought out and investigated for appropriateness and suitability. For example, a massage therapist, reiki practitioner, nature therapist or gymnasium coach.

The study suggests that MHPs should trust and have confidence in any referring professionals when sending clients to try an additional co-occurring therapy. It is crucial that MHPs thoroughly investigate the referred professionals to avoid making the wrong recommendation. If this is not undertaken, and the client's expectations are not met, a breach of trust may be experienced by the survivor, potentially harming the therapeutic relationship and trust between the MHP and the survivor. Such mistakes could potentially cause further harm and re-traumatise clients. These studies recommend a collaborative and empathetic therapeutic approach, informed by evidence-based treatment models and holistic therapies, to help survivors regain their sense of self-worth, develop healthy boundaries, create new trusted connections, and cultivate self-compassion.

Ethical Dilemma

These studies report an ethical and contentious dilemma regarding the lack of education MHPs have to treat survivors. This dilemma was described by survivors as the MHPs working outside their level of expertise and, in some cases, causing further harm to them by not understanding them, stopping treatment and referring survivors to other MHPs. Termination of therapy conveyed a negative message, reinforcing survivors' beliefs about themselves as having no hope and no one to help, which exacerbated their feelings of abandonment. Further consequences of this unexpected termination of treatment for survivors included pre-empting the therapist terminating the session by dropping out or ending the therapy themselves, resulting in some survivors giving up treatment altogether. In addition, some survivors reported that paying for unhelpful treatments left them frustrated and out of pocket.

Health Literacy

These studies reported on the extensive health literacy of survivors, with 30 references from six participants recorded on various topics such as boundaries, identity, and trauma-informed care. The traits identified are commonly associated with suicidal behaviours, highlighting the need for increased awareness and support for survivors. Identifying these traits indicates a need for expanded SPA psychoeducation programs for both MHPs and survivors to raise awareness of the lasting effects of child abuse trauma. These studies suggest that high literacy levels were driven by the survivors' need to understand their trauma. High literacy levels in survivors are an area proposed for further investigation.

Mental Health and Identity

These studies highlight the significant impact of CITs on survivors. The participants shared their struggles with mental health conditions such as anxiety, depression, complex post-traumatic stress disorder, dissociation, and emotional attachment disorder. The study also revealed the connection between identity and suicidality, with some participants feeling trapped in the narratives imposed on them by the AP as children. In addition, the effects of enmeshment and brainwashing were present in many participants, leaving them feeling unsafe, suicidal, and with no sense of identity.

The complexity and depth of thought that goes into planning to die by suicide due to lifelong narratives being told to one survivor by his AP highlights the urgent need for trauma-informed therapy. These studies recommend that MHPs understand the intergenerational effects of SPA, the impact of enmeshment and brainwashing, and the connection between identity and suicidality. The study also highlights the importance of empowering survivors to reclaim their identities and break free from the narratives imposed upon them as children.

Different Sides of Suicide

The results of these studies shed light on the significant impact of suicide on survivors who have experienced suicidal ideation or have had a family member die by suicide due to SPA. The findings of these studies revealed that 50% of the survivors identified that they had thought about and planned to die by suicide; however, they stopped before completion. Furthermore, 30% of the survivors mentioned that they had thought about suicide but would not act impulsively. In addition, two participants feel that they often have to support their siblings to prevent them from dying by suicide due to SPA. These figures highlight the importance of providing high-quality mental health support to survivors to help them cope with their experiences and prevent the risk of suicide completion. These studies recommend implementing trauma-informed suicide prevention measures and interventions as a crucial step to addressing this significant issue. MHPs need to be trained to recognise and respond to suicide risk factors such as unresolved CIT experiences in survivors to prevent suicide completion.

Identity and Brainwashing

These studies reported the significant impact of enmeshment and brainwashing on survivors' identity and mental health. Participants spoke of the need to appease their AP, which left them feeling unsafe, suicidal, and without a clear sense of identity. They were not allowed to be anything but what their AP wanted. The connection between identity and suicidality was highlighted by several participants, with one sharing the difficulty of living with the engraved pain of childhood SPA trauma. These studies recommend promoting healthy relationships and addressing the cognitive dissonance and suicidal ideation experienced by survivors.

Early research on PA indicates that emotional manipulation strategies, brainwashing techniques, and the programming of children are common elements of parental alienation (Baker, 2007). These studies' results report that survivors of SPA feel as though they were brainwashed and unable to reverse the damage caused by these techniques. In addition, the survivor participants in these studies spoke about the manipulative brainwashing techniques used to invoke fear, persuade, control, and manipulate them as children, many of whom have not recovered. These findings are noteworthy since previous research has been limited regarding whether survivors still feel the effects of brainwashing from their childhoods and if they ever find a way to recover from the techniques used to alienate them from their TPs (Baker, 2007).

Parent Threatening Suicide to Control the Survivor

These studies highlight the devastating impact that the threat of suicide can have on individuals, particularly when used as a tool for control or manipulation by their AP. For example, the findings suggest that one of the survivor study participants experienced significant emotional trauma due to his mother threatening suicide when he asked about his father. These ongoing experiences have had a lasting impact on their ability to trust and form relationships. Moreover, these studies highlight the importance of developing a strong sense of self-agency in adulthood, which is crucial in overcoming feelings of powerlessness and developing healthy self-esteem. By recognising the damaging effects of suicide threats and taking steps to promote healthy relationships and self-agency, MHPs can work towards preventing the harmful impact of these experiences on individuals and communities.

Furthermore, these studies emphasise the need to raise awareness about the long-term effects of suicide on survivors and the importance of preventing SPA. These studies also report that survivors of false allegations may feel stigmatised and isolated, with some hiding their childhood experiences from their partners and children out of shame and embarrassment. Additionally, when survivors confront the accuser about the false allegations, it can be an emotional and difficult process, with the accuser feeling defensive and unwilling to admit the allegations were false, exacerbating feelings of betrayal and anger in the survivor as the drawing out of unresolved trauma. These studies recommend that MHPs be aware of the stigmatisation and isolation that survivors may have experienced and provide support and validation to help them navigate these challenges. Furthermore, it is important to raise awareness within the Family Court system about the impact of false allegations of CSA on survivors and their TPs to prevent these experiences from perpetuating trauma within the survivors' community.

False Allegations of Child Sexual Abuse and Family Court

These studies report that false allegations of child CSA for survivors who had been through the Family Court system as children of PA and SPA were found to have a significant long-term impact on their adverse emotional and physical reactions due to CITs. Other reported emotions were persistent betrayal, shame, compound grief, loss, lack of recognition, extreme anger, depression, anxiety, bulimia, migraines, and CPTSD. Furthermore, one survivor whose TP was accused of perpetrating CSA with her spoke of the shame and embarrassment that followed her throughout the Court experience as a child and into her adult life due to the Courts believing the AP and not believing her or her TP. The survivor also spoke of her AP getting the FDV and Court workers to align against the TP and how she could not stop it due to not being recognised as credible once they started blaming the TP. This survivor also warned of the lifelong shame and humiliation of a sexually based incestual crime that was never committed.

Furthermore, the survivor shared that the community she lived in at the time all knew about the allegations of CSA aimed at her TP, and now she feels stigmatised for life and is known as the adult child who had sex with their own parent. She explained that this can never be undone and should never have happened in the first place. She also stated that the professional FDV workers, solicitors and the Magistrate in Court should have had more training.

This survivor shared, "It all could have been prevented if they understood the dynamics of SPA and how you cannot identify the truth if you are not trained to recognise SPA symptoms in a child and their TP." This participant cried throughout the interview and stated that she feels she will never recover from what happened to her or her TP in Family Court. This participant also reported that as an adult with children, her AP aligned with her ex-husband and took her children off her, again with false allegations of abuse against her toward the child this time. Furthermore, the AP wanted full custody of the adult survivor's own child, her grandchild. These studies report that the repeat PABs of an AP can carry through to the next generation and were not noticed in Family Court all these years later. These studies recommend the urgent need for legal professionals to receive training on the dynamics of SPA and the long-term effects of false allegations of CSA on survivors.

SPA and Abduction

These studies shed light on the often-overlooked issue of SPA and child abduction (SPAA) during divorce and separation and its long-term effects on survivors. Three interviews with survivor participants revealed that their SPA child abductions were a complex and deeply traumatic event that went unnoticed, unacknowledged, and unreported by members of their own communities, such as teachers, Police, medical personnel and family friends. In addition, the data highlighted that SPAA does have significant consequences on survivors' mental health, trust, identity, and ability to adapt to new situations. Moreover, the study revealed that SPAA is relatively common and has historically been covered up by the narrative that the 'relationship broke down, and the other parent and kids just moved out'.

Survivor participants in these studies reported that some parents believe it is their right to move a child away from their schools, family, and friends and away from their beloved parent. Data reported that this belief is harmful and profoundly misguided. Survivor participants explained that they were moved away, also described as abducted by survivors, to another town, interstate or internationally. According to the study participants who experienced SPAA, their parents did not consider moving a child without consent as abduction. Survivors suggested that they wanted the Family Court to have this psychologically abusive abduction narrative and action immediately stopped and changed.

Furthermore, the SPAA survivors assert that moving a child without consent should be considered a criminal act that should not be undertaken at any point unless there is police and protective services involvement and substantiated abuse. The survivor study participants shared that none of them will ever get over their experiences of SPAA and hope that the laws will change around taking children away from safe, loving parents. In addition, participants shared their experiences of grandparent and relative alienation after child abduction occurred, which the survivors reported was just as detrimental to them as abduction itself.

The study also highlighted the financial burden of bringing a child back after an abduction, the extensive court process, the psychological harm it does to the child at the time, and how it affects their adulthood. Furthermore, there are few sanctions for parents who commit SPAA, which is a significant concern for survivors in these studies. Given the repercussions described by the survivors, there is a need for legal and policy frameworks to protect children from these traumatic experiences.

These studies recommend that parents should not be allowed to take children without the other parent (the TP) or the TP's extended families' knowledge. Also recommended is that a court of law never approves a move away from the child's TP. The study participants reported that in Australia's SPA and child abduction cases, the Police do not get involved as they consider this a Family Court matter, not a child abduction matter. The participants were adamant that they want this legislation changed to stop SPAA from occurring so that all children can have access to safe and loving parents and extended family members to live fulfilling lives. The study's findings recommend that the laws around taking children away from safe, loving parents must be changed immediately to prevent future cases of SPAA.

Physical Health

These studies reported the physical health conditions offered by six of the eleven survivors' and one MHP's data. These conditions were offered without prompting, and due to these unexpected contributions and the current lack of research in this area, they were included and compared to previously collated research from other studies on the physical health challenges of adult trauma survivors. Within these studies' data, the 28 new health conditions reported by survivors differed from the previous data describing 13 health challenges survivors might develop (Downey et al., 2017; Felitti et al., 1998; Perry, 2003). These health conditions were not investigated further in these studies.

Notably, 30% of the study participants reported receiving a formal medical diagnosis for their physical symptoms. The health challenges the remaining 70% of the survivors described were their perceptions and may be subjective as data was not obtained regarding whether a medical professional confirmed their diagnosis. This offering of information highlights more significant health concerns about the extent to which survivors may be living with undiagnosed physical health conditions related to their experiences of childhood abuse. This is particularly concerning given the high prevalence of physical health challenges reported in these studies and previous research among survivors of childhood abuse and SPA.

The physical health challenges reported by the survivors in these studies highlight the need for MHPs to work closely with survivors and their medical teams to address the physical symptoms that may be linked to their experiences of childhood abuse. In addition, these studies recommend that MHPs collaborate with medical professionals to ensure survivors receive comprehensive care that addresses their mental and physical health needs. Further research is needed to understand these comorbid conditions' underlying mechanisms and develop targeted interventions. Moreover, the presence of five reported cases of cancer and one case of leukaemia by the MHP participant in a shared workplace suggests that practitioners may be at risk for some cancers, although the specific types were not described in these studies.

Significant Clinical Findings of the Research-Specific Phobia-Severe Parental Alienation and Abduction Anxiety Variant

These studies found that three out of four survivors who had experienced SPAA as children under eight shared similar experiences and emotions with the Practitioner-Researcher, leading the Researcher to uncover a new anxiety variant that has not been researched before. This finding is noteworthy, given the dearth of research on the impact of SPAA on children under eight, particularly concerning specific phobias. While other sources may have covered this topic previously, the Researcher came across only one source in the published grey literature that explored the anxiety variant associated with SPAA in children under eight.

It is crucial to emphasise that the Researcher's personal experience with a specific phobia played a significant role in uncovering this discovery. Due to having experienced specific phobia firsthand, the Researcher could identify its presence in survivors of SPAA. This underscores the significance of personal experiences when exploring new aspects of child abuse trauma. When practitioners possess a unique understanding of trauma, they are better equipped to recognise symptoms and offer practical support to those impacted.

Survivor Challenges and Resilience

These studies report that the lived experience of SPA was varied and unique for each participant. While many survivors experienced overwhelming challenges growing up as children of SPA and SPAA, they developed diverse adaptation methods, including personal resilience, coping styles, and protective self-care factors. Others developed differently, such as observing and comparing their methods and copying other community members. However, the road to acceptance has been difficult for many survivors, and these challenges and CITs are what MHPs need to recognise.

These studies highlight the urgent need for MHPs to understand, recognise and successfully treat survivors. The participants shared 211 individual references, with a significant undercurrent theme emphasising the importance of their experiences being heard and understood. The excerpts presented in these studies provide powerful insights into the mind of a severely alienated adult survivor, with the survivors hoping that by sharing these highly personal experiences, MHPs will gain a deeper understanding of their trauma and consequently learn a new way to work with them that is holistic as well as based on previous trauma-informed research. Ultimately, the goal is to provide survivors with the support and resources they need to heal and overcome the lasting impact of SPA.

Limitations of the Study

Sample Size

The Researcher identified several limitations in the study involving survivors. Firstly, the sample size of survivors and MHP participants was relatively small, with only twenty-one individuals included. A larger sample size would benefit future research, allowing for more robust findings.

Insider Researcher

Another limitation acknowledged by the Researcher was the potential bias of being an insider researcher. Being intimately familiar with the subject matter of SPA, there was a risk of making assumptions or drawing conclusions based on pre-existing knowledge. To address this limitation, the Researcher remained aware of her role as a researcher throughout the data collection process. She consciously avoided letting her personal experiences or professional background influence the interviews, constantly focusing on the research objectives.

Additionally, throughout the data collection phase, the Researcher kept a diary regarding any emotional triggers that may have been affected by listening to survivor accounts but not being able to counsel them or stop their trauma. This part of the research was complex because the survivors knew that the Researcher had lived experience herself and was an MHP and wanted to tell the Researcher about everything that had happened to them so they could connect with someone who understood their trauma. For some, this was the first time they had told their story to anyone. Unfortunately, the Researcher could not engage them in that manner as she needed to retain her position as a researcher, not an MHP.

Advantages of the Research

The Researcher notes that the survivor's knowing she had lived the experience of SPAA and was an MHP was also an advantage. The

Researcher discovered this as the survivors shared that they felt very comfortable with her and divulged information they had never read about or shared with anyone. This deep level of trust and extensive sharing was reflected in the research data, which contributed to new information in these studies that had not been recorded before. In addition, the survivors made a point that as emotional as the interviews were for many of them, they wanted the world to understand their pain and the MHPs to deeply understand them and create a protocol to help them heal if they come forward.

Physical Health Accounts are Not Proven

Another limitation noted was that none of the physical health accounts offered by the survivors was medically proven by a professional to associate their child abuse recounts directly with SPA. One reason these survivor accounts may not have been formally agreed upon ties into the study's results, reporting a substantial lack of MHP and community professionals trained to identify CITs in the area of SPA in the community. At this point in the research, where there is still a lack of validated research linking CITs with SPA, it would be prudent for the research and medical fields to listen to survivor accounts, realisations, and stories of why and when symptoms started manifesting. However, survivors' intuitive beliefs and conclusions about their psychological and physical health, when their symptoms started, and why are strong arguments to contest due to limited research.

Future Directions in SPA Research

Inclusion of Lived Experience Practitioner-Researchers

For MHPs to improve the care and support for survivors of SPA, further research is necessary to explore different areas of this complex issue. Including adult survivor practitioner-researchers in future studies on SPA is imperative because their lived experiences can provide valuable insights into the complex and sensitive issues surrounding SPA abuse. By incorporating their perspectives, researchers can gain a deeper understanding of the impact of SPA on survivors, leading to more effective interventions and support and staying true to the motto, 'nothing about us without us.'

Inclusion of Lived Experience Indigenous Practitioner-Researchers

Similarly, when Indigenous Australian SPA studies are undertaken, it is important to include Indigenous people on the research team because they uniquely understand their cultural practices, beliefs, and unique experiences (Australian Institute of Aboriginal and Torres Strait Islander Studies, 2012). Including indigenous people in research can ensure that cultural sensitivities are respected and that research findings are more accurate, relevant, and meaningful (Australian Institute of Aboriginal and Torres Strait Islander Studies, 2012). This approach is consistent with the principles of decolonising research, which seeks to challenge and transform the power dynamics inherent in the research and promote the agency of indigenous people (Australian Human Rights Commission, 1997). In both cases, including the perspectives of those with lived experience can lead to more authentic and honest data that can be used to create new and effective interventions and support services for survivors while staying true to the motto, 'nothing about us without us.'

Development of Evidence-Based Guidelines

Moreover, future research should focus on developing evidence-based guidelines for MHPs and policymakers to address survivors' challenges and improve their mental health outcomes. The diverse range of physical conditions reported in these studies also highlights the need for further research to understand the impact of childhood trauma on physical health and develop appropriate interventions to support survivors.

Inclusion in Decision-Making Processes

These studies also recommend that professionals within the SPA field actively involve survivors in the future direction of decision-making processes while recognising their perspectives as valuable. In addition, PA organisations can make a more contemporary contribution by including survivors in research, symposiums, advocacy, and PA organisations. This approach would be more inclusive and collaborative, reflecting survivors and their families' needs and experiences.

Future research should explore the potential contributions of adult SPA survivors in the SPA field apart from being study participants (not taking away from the survivors who are studying PA and in advocacy and support group roles at present). The present study suggests that these survivors have unique insights and lived experiences that can inform policy and practice regarding SPA. However, further research is needed to determine the most effective ways to involve survivors in decision-making processes and ensure their perspectives are valued. Additionally, more research is required to investigate the best approaches to providing support and resources for survivors.

Payment for Research

The Researcher suggests that payment for research does not occur as APs sometimes use this method to create enmeshment with the survivors as a child, which may, in turn, develop a level of re-victimisation. Payment or gifts may also have been bestowed upon children of SPA to maintain power and control over the child for the perpetrator's personal gain. These studies illustrate that MHPs should try to be safe and predictable, unlike the AP, when working with survivors.

These studies also recommend that further research be undertaken to develop effective interventions to address the long-term effects of brainwashing and thought reform experienced by survivors of SPA. This recommendation is necessary because, as highlighted in these studies, survivors still feel the effects of brainwashing from their childhoods. Many have not recovered from the techniques used to manipulate and control them by their AP. Some survivors report that they are still being manipulated by their AP even in their fifties and sixties. MHPs need to learn about cults, brainwashing, thought reform and how to undo it as part of their professional development and clinical supervision.

Final Note from the Author Regarding Publishing a PhD in Book Form

In the pioneering realm of adult survivors of child psychological abuse research and the dedicated mental health and law professionals who navigate this terrain, conflict is not just prevalent, it is ubiquitous. Parents are embroiled in battles for custody, experts spar over research methodologies, terminologies, and affiliations, while the children and adult survivors observe from the shadows. However, this status quo is poised for a transformative shift.

As a recent PhD recipient immersed in the pioneering field of SPA research and therapeutic intervention, I confront a formidable hurdle: the exorbitant publishing fees that now loom ominously over academia. Even with the involvement of PhD supervisors and PA experts in co-authoring publications from the twin PhD, we faced hurdles in getting them published, indicating the complexity and difficulties in navigating the process. I am now at a crossroads no longer shielded by the read-and-publish agreements afforded to PhD candidates.

By opting for a book format, I could present my findings comprehensively, weaving together diverse content and insights that the limitations of journal articles might have constrained. Moreover, books offer a longer shelf life, ensuring that my research remains accessible and relevant to academic and practitioner audiences for years to come. This approach aligns with my goal of making meaningful contributions to the field while navigating the challenges of limited resources. Additionally, the expedited publication process of a book allows for quicker dissemination of crucial information, potentially saving lives by providing timely insights for mental health practitioners to understand better and support adult survivors of trauma.

Could this be the harbinger of a new era in academic publishing? A paradigm shift where scholars reclaim control over their narratives, unencumbered by prohibitive publishing fees? The resonance of this decision extends far beyond my individual circumstances—it signals a rallying cry for academics worldwide who refuse to be shackled by the confines of traditional publishing models. It's a clarion call for innovation, inclusivity, and accessibility in scholarly dissemination. I dream of a future where knowledge knows no bounds and voices previously marginalised find their rightful place in the academic discourse.

References

ACES Too High News. (2020, May 20). Retrieved from ACES Too High: https://acestoohigh.com/got-your-ace-score/

Adams, S. A., & Riggs, S. A. (2008). An exploratory study of vicarious trauma among therapist trainees. *Training and Education in Professional Psychology, 2*(1), 26-34. doi:https://doi-org.ezproxy.usc.edu.au/10.1037/1931-3918.2.1.26

Ahrens, C. E., Stansell, J., & Jennings, A. (2010). To Tell or Not to Tell: The Impact of Disclosure on Sexual Assault Survivors' Recovery. *Violence and Victims, 25*(5), 631-648. Retrieved February February 11, 2023, 2023, from https://www.proquest.com/docview/817785178?accountid=28745&parentSessionId=lpvSLwjyUL7haPMlMTSKxRf1N5x-8WuCHxrZf1IUOlbU%3D&pq-origsite=primo

Alaggia, R. (2010, February). An Ecological Analysis of Child Sexual Abuse Disclosure: Considerations for Child and Adolescent Mental Health. *Journal of the Canadian Academy of Child and Adolescent Psychiatry, 19*(1), 23-39. Retrieved February 11, 2023, from https://www.ncbi.nlm.nih.gov/pmc/articles/PMC2809444/

Alder, C., & Polk, K. (2001). *Child Victims of Homicide.* Cambridge: Cambridge University Press.

Alexander, P. C. (2015). *Intergenerational Cycles of Trauma and Violence. An Attachment and Family Systems Perspective* (1 ed.). New York, NY, America: W.W Norton & Company Inc.

Alvarez, M., & Turner, C. (ND). *About Us.* Retrieved from Resetting the Family: https://www.resetting-the-family.com/

American Cancer Society. (2023). *Cancer Clusters.* Retrieved June 30, 2023, from American Cancer Society: https://www.cancer.org/cancer/risk-prevention/understanding-cancer-risk/cancer-clusters.html

American Cancer Society. (2023, June 30). *Do X-rays and Gamma Rays Cause Cancer?* Retrieved 2023, from American Cancer Society: https://www.cancer.org/cancer/risk-prevention/radiation-exposure/x-rays-gamma-rays/do-xrays-and-gamma-rays-cause-cancer.html

American Psychiatric Association. (2013). *Diagnostic and Statistical Manual of Mental Disorders DSM-5* (5 ed.). Arlington, VA, USA: American Psychiatric Publishing. Retrieved October 238, 2021

American Psychiatric Association. (2013). *Diagnostics and Statistical Manual of Mental Disorders* (5 ed.). Arlington, Virginia, America: American Psychiatric Publishing. Retrieved November 1, 2020

American Psychological Association. (2020). *APA Dictionary of Psychology.* Retrieved June 23, 2020, from American Psychological Association: https://dictionary.apa.org/psychodynamic-theory

American Psychological Association. (2021, June). *Carl Rogers, PhD. 1947 APA President.* Retrieved April 10, 2023, from American Psychological Association: https://www.apa.org/about/governance/president/carl-r-rogers

Anand, K. S., & Dhikav, V. (2012, Oct-Dec). Hippocampus in health and disease: An overview. *Annals of Indian Academy of Neurology, 15*(4), 239-246. doi: 10.4103/0972-2327.104323

Anderson, C. A., & Bushman, B. J. (2002, February 1). Human Aggression. *Annual Review of Psychology, 53*(1), 27-51. doi:10.1146/annurev.psych.53.100901.135231

Andrews, T. (2012). What is Social Constructionism? *The Grounded Theory Review, 11*(1), 39-46. Retrieved March 12, 2023, from https://web-p-ebscohost-com.ezproxy.usc.edu.au/ehost/pdfviewer/pdfviewer?vid=1&sid=e45494c5-4762-4104-9622-f384ee8528f9%40redis

Arksey, H., & O'Malley, L. (2003). Scoping studies: towards a methodological framework. *International Journal of Social Research Methodology, 8*(1), 19-32. doi:doi-org.ezproxy.usc.edu.au/10.1080/1364557032000119616

Australian Government. (2019, November 27). *Marriages and Divorces, Australia.* Retrieved July 26, 2021, from Australian Bureau of Statistics: https://www.abs.gov.au/statistics/people/people-and-communities/marriages-and-divorces-australia/latest-release

Australian Government. (2022, November 17). *What is family and domestic violence?* Retrieved January 14, 2023, from Services Australia:

https://www.servicesaustralia.gov.au/what-family-and-domestic-violence?context=60033

Australian Human Rights Commission. (1997). *Bringing Them Home.* Canberra: Commonwealth of Australia. Retrieved January 17, 2021, from https://humanrights.gov.au/our-work/bringing-them-home-report-1997

Australian Institute of Aboriginal and Torres Strait Islander Studies. (2012). *Guidelines for Ethical Research in Australian Indigenous Studies.* AIATSIS. Australian Institute of Aboriginal and Torres Strait Islander Studies. Retrieved August 17, 2023, from https://aiatsis.gov.au/sites/default/files/2020-09/gerais.pdf

Australian Institute of Health and Welfare. (2018-2019, March 18). *Child Protection Australia 2018-19: children in the child protection system.* Retrieved February 9, 2021, from Australian Institute of Health and Welfare: https://www.aihw.gov.au/reports/child-protection/child-protection-australia-children-in-the-child-protection-system/contents/children-in-substantiated-cases-of-abuse-or-neglect

Bahtiyar, S., Karaca, K. G., Henckens, M. J., & Roozendaal, B. (2020, October). Norepinephrine and glucocorticoid effects on the brain mechanisms underlying memory accuracy and generalization. *Molecular and Cellular Neuroscience, 108*, 1-10. doi:https://doi.org/10.1016/j.mcn.2020.103537

Baker, A. (1994, January). The cult of parenthood: A qualitative study of parental alienation. *Cultic Studies Review, 4*(1), 20. Retrieved February 15, 2021, from Research Gate: https://www.researchgate.net/publication/228344114_The_cult_of_parenthood_A_qualitative_study_of_parental_alienation

Baker, A. J. (2006). Patterns of Parental Alienation Syndrome: A Qualitative Study of Adults Who were Alienated from a Parent as a Child. *American Journal of Family Therapy, 34*(1), 63-78. doi:10.1080/01926180500301444

Baker, A. J. (2007). *Adult Children of Parental Alienation Syndrome. Breaking the Ties that Bind.* New York, New York, USA: W.W Norton & Company. Retrieved November 7, 2020

Baker, A. J. (2007). *Adult Children of Parental Alienation Syndrome. Breaking the Ties that Bind.* New York, New York, USA: W.W Norton & Company. Retrieved November 7, 2020

Baker, A. J., & Chambers, J. (2011, January 7). Adult Recall of Childhood Exposure to Parental Conflict: Unpacking the Black Box of Parental Alienation. *Journal of Divorce and Remarriage, 52*(1), 55-76. doi:10.1080/10502556.2011.534396

Baker, A. J., & Fine, P. R. (2014). *Surviving Parental Alienation: A Journey of Hope and Healing.* Lanham, Maryland, USA: Rowman & Littlefield.

Baker, A. J., & Schneiderman, M. (2015). Bonded to the Abuser. How victims make sense of the abuse. London, England: Rowman & Littlefield.

Baker, A. J., & Verrocchio, C. (2014, December 25). Parental Bonding and Parental Alienation as Correlates of Psychological Maltreatment in Adults in Intact and Non-intact Families. *Journal of Child and Family Studies, 24*, 3047-3057. doi:DOI 10.1007/s10826-014-0108-0

Baker, A. J., & Verrocchio, M. C. (2013, November 13). Italian College Student-Reported Childhood Exposure to Parental Alienation: Correlates With Well-Being. *Journal of Divorce & Remarriage, 54*(8), 609-628. doi:10.1080/10502556.2013.837714

Baker, A. J., Fine, P. R., & Lacheen-Baker, A. (2020). *Restoring Family Connections.* Lanham, Maryland, USA: Rowman & Littlefield. Retrieved January 28, 2022

Barnett, J. E., & Coffman, C. (2015, June). *Termination and Abandonment. A Proactive Approach to Ethical Practice.* Retrieved June 7, 2021, from Society for the Advancement of Psychotherapy: www.societyforpsychotherapy.org/termination-and-abandonment-a-proactive-approach-to-ethical-practice

Bentley, C., & Matthewson, M. (2020). The Not-Forgotten Child: Alienated Adult Children's Experience of Parental Alienation. *The American Journal of Family Therapy, 48*(5), 509-529. doi:https://www.tandfonline.com/doi/full/10.1080/01926187.2020.1775531

Bergen, R. K. (1993). Interviewing survivors of marital rape: Doing feminist research on sensitive topics. In *Researching Sensitive Topics* (pp. 197-211). Newbury Park, California, USA: Sage.

Berkowitz, A. R. (n.d). *Parental Alienation Syndrome.* Retrieved June 26, 2021, from Dr Alice R Berkowitz: https://www.draliceberkowitz.com/alienation

Bernet, W. (2008, October 13). Parental Alienation Disorder and DSM-V. *The American Journal of Family Therapy, 36*(5), 349-366. doi:https://doi.org/10.1080/01926180802405513

Bernet, W. (2010). *Parental Alienation, DSM-5, and ICD-11.* Springfield, Illinois, USA: Charles C Thomas.

Blakely, L. (2022, February 21). Learning to Become a More Ethically Focused Practitioner Researcher: Developing Through the Research Ethics Process. *Ethics and Social Welfare, 16*(3), 322-331. doi:https://doi-org.ezproxy.usc.edu.au/10.1080/17496535.2022.2033397

Boonzaier, F., & de la Rey, C. (2004, September 1). Woman Abuse: The Construction of Gender in Women and Men's Narratives of Violence. *South African Journal of Psychology, 34*(3), 443-463. doi:https://doi-org.ezproxy.usc.edu.au/10.1177/008124630403400307

Boswell, E., & Babchuk, W. (2022). Philosophical and theoretical underpinnings of qualitative research. In *INTERNATIONAL ENCYLOPEDIA OF EDUCATION* (pp. 1-13). Lincoln, NE, America. doi:DOI:10.1016/b978-0-12-818630-5.11001-2

Bourget, D., Grace, J., & Whitehurst, L. (2007, March). A Review of Maternal and Paternal Filicide. *The Journal of the American Academy of Psychiatry and the Law, 35*(1), 74-82. Retrieved May 28, 2023, from https://jaapl.org/content/35/1/74.long

Bourne, E. J. (1998). *Overcoming Specific Phobia. A Hierarchy and Exposure-Based Protocol for the Treatment of All Specific Phobias.* (C. Honeychurch, Ed.) Oakland, California, United States: Publisher's West Group.

Bowlby, J. (1980). *Loss, Sadness and Depression* (Vol. 3). New York, New York, America: The Travistock Institute of Human Resources.

Bowlby, J. (1988). *A Secure Base: Clinical Applications of Attachment Theory.* New York: Brunner-Routledge.

Boyatzis, R. E. (1998). *Transforming Qualitative Information.* London: SAGE Publications.

Braun, V., & Clarke, V. (2006). Using thematic analysis in psychology. *Qualitative Research in Psychology, 3*(2), 77-101. doi:10.1191/1478088706qp063oa

Braun, V., & Clarke, V. (2014, October 16). What can "thematic analysis" offer health and wellbeing researchers? *International Journal of Qualitative Studies in Health and Well-being, 9*(10), 1-3. doi:10.3402/qhw.v9.26152

Briere, J. N. (1992). *Child Abuse Trauma.* Southern California, USA: Sage Publications Inc.

Briere, J., & Runtz, M. (1987). Post Sexual Abuse Trauma: Data and Implications for Clinical Practice. *Journal of Interpersonal Violence, 2*(4), 376-379. doi:https://doi-org.ezproxy.usc.edu.au/10.1177/088626058700200403

Briere, J., & Runtz, M. (1993, September 1). Childhood Sexual Abuse Long term Sequelae and Implications for Psychological Assessment. *Journal of Interpersonal Violence, 8*(3), 312-330. doi:https://doi-org.ezproxy.usc.edu.au/10.1177/088626093008003002

Briere, J., & Spinazzola, J. (2005). Phenomenology and psychological assessment of complex trauma states. *Journal of Traumatic Stress, 18*(5), 401-412. doi:DOI:10.1002/jts.20048

Britannica Dictionary. (2023). *Homicide-Law.* Retrieved from Britannica: https://www.britannica.com/biography/Richard-Ramirez

Brown, D. P., & Elliot, D. S. (2016). *Attachment Disturbances in Adults. Treatment for Comprehensive Repair* (Vol. One). New York, New York, America: W W Norton and Company, Inc. Retrieved October 8, 2022

Brown, T., Tyson, D., & Arias, P. F. (2014, April 16). Filicide and Parental Separation and Divorce. *Child Abuse Review. Association of Child Protection Professionals, 23*, 79-88. doi:10.1002/car.2327

Bruce, T. J., & Sanderson, W. C. (1998). *Specific Phobias, Clinical Applications of Evidence Based Psychotherapy.* (R. D. Hack, Ed.) Montebello, NY, United States: Book-mart Press.

Bryant, A., & Charmaz, K. (2007). *The SAGE Handbook of Grounded Theory.* London: SAGE Publications Ltd.

Burr, V. (2003). *Social Constructionism* (2 ed.). New York, NY, USA: Routledge.

Butz, M. R., & Evans, F. (2019). Factitious Disorder by Proxy, Parent Alienation, and the Argument for Interrelated Multidimensional Diagnoses. *Professional Psychology: Research and Practice, 50*(6), 364-375. doi:https://doi-org.ezproxy.usc.edu.au/10.1037/pro0000250

Cahill, L., & Alkire, M. (2003, March). Epinephrine enhancement of human memory consolidation: Interaction with arousal at encoding. *Neurobiology of Learning and Memory, 79*(2), 194-198. doi:https://doi.org/10.1016/S1074-7427(02)00036-9

Campbell, C., & Clarke, M. (2019, July 18). The 'Worker-Researcher': Introducing a new interview dynamic. *Qualitative Research in Psychology, 19*(2), 405-423. doi:https://doi-org.ezproxy.usc.edu.au/10.1080/14780887.2019.1644408

Canadian Center for Occupational Health and Safety. (2023, June 13). *Occupational Cancer.* Retrieved June 30, 2023, from Canadian Center for Occupational Health and Safety: https://www.ccohs.ca/oshanswers/diseases/cancer/occupational_cancer.html#:~:text=The%20most%20common%20types%20of,cancer%2C%20bladder%20cancer%20and%20mesothelioma.&text=*%20In%20general%2C%20the%20overall%20attributable,risk%20may%20be%20around%2090%25.

Carpenter, L. L., Tyrka, A. R., Ross, N. S., Khoury, L., Anderson, G. M., & Price, L. H. (2009, July 1). Effect of Childhood Emotional Abuse and Age on Cortisol Responsivity in Adulthood. *Biological Psychiatry, 66*(1), 69-75. doi:https://doi.org/10.1016/j.biopsych.2009.02.030

Cashmore, J., & Shackel, R. (2013, January). *The long-term effects of child sexual abuse.* Retrieved May 19, 2023, from Australian Government. Australian Institue of Family Studies: https://aifs.gov.au/resources/policy-and-practice-papers/long-term-effects-child-sexual-abuse

Centers for Disease Control and Prevention. (2019). *Marriage and Divorce.* Retrieved July 26, 2021, from National Centers for Disease Control and Prevention: https://www.cdc.gov/nchs/fastats/marriage-divorce.htm

Centers for Disease Control and Prevention. (2020, April 20). *Violence Prevention.* Retrieved February 15, 2021, from Centers for Disease Control and Prevention: https://www.cdc.gov/violenceprevention/aces/fastfact.html?CDC_AA_refVal=https%3A%2F%2Fwww.cdc.gov-%2Fviolenceprevention%2Facestudy%2Ffastfact.html

Chamberlin, J. (2015, April). Are your clients leaving too soon? *American Psychological Association, 46*(4), 1-5. Retrieved December 4, 2022, from https://www.apa.org/monitor/2015/04/clients

Charmaz, K. (2014). *Constructing Grounded Theory* (2 ed.). Sage Publications.

Childress, C. (2014, December 4). Treatment of Attachment-Based "Parental Alienation". *CalSouthern Psychology.* California, America. Retrieved June 17, 2021, from https://www.youtube.com/watch?v=ezBJ3954mKw

Childress, C. A. (2015). *Foundations.* Claremont, California, America: Oaksong Press. Retrieved October 31, 2020

Childress, C. A. (2022). *Child Custody Evaluations.* Retrieved January 30, 2022, from Dr Craig A Childress: https://drcachildress.org/custom-page/6-child-custody-evaluations/

Childress, C. A. (2022). *The Office of Dr C.A. Childress.* Retrieved January 30, 2022, from Dr C.A Childress: https://drcachildress.org/

Chorpita, B. F., Albano, A., & Barlow, D. H. (2010, June 7). Child Anxiety Sensitivity Index: Considerations for Children with Anxiety Disorders. *Journal of Clinical Child Psychology, 25*(1), 77-82. doi:https://doi-org.ezproxy.usc.edu.au/10.1207/s15374424jccp2501_9

Clawar, S. S., & Rivlin, B. V. (2014). *Children Held Hostage: Identifying Brainwashed Children, Presenting a Case, and Crafting Solutions.* Chicago, Illinois, America: American Bar Association.

Cleary, R., & Armour, C. (2022, July 29). Exploring the role of practitioner lived experience of mental health issues in counselling and psychotherapy. *Counselling and Psychotherapy Research, 22*(4), 1100-1111. doi:https://doi.org/10.1002/capr.12569

Cleary, R., & Armour, C. (2022, July 29). Exploring the role of practitioner lived experience of mental health issues in counselling and psychotherapy. *Counselling and Psychotherapy Research, 22*(4), 1100-1111. doi: https://doi.org/10.1002/capr.12569

Coan, J. A. (2008). *Toward a neuroscience of attachment: Theory, research, and clinical applications.* New York, America: Guildford.

Collins Dictionary. (2023). *Definition of familicide.* Retrieved January 14, 2023, from Collins Dictionary: https://www.collinsdictionary.com/dictionary/english/familicide

Collins-Mrakas, A. (2004). *Guidelines for Conducting Research with People who are Homeless.* Retrieved Nov 13, 2015, from York University: http://www.yorku.ca/research/documents/2010Guidelines%20-%20Research%20with%20People%20who%20are%20Homeless.doc

Conscious Co-Parenting Institute. (2022). *Conscious Co-Parenting Institute Hits New Milestone During Pandemic.* Retrieved January 13, 2022, from Conscious Co-Parenting Institute: https://www.consciouscoparentinginstitute.com/conscious-co-parenting-institute-hits-new-milestone-during-pandemic/

Conscious Co-Parenting Institute. (2022). *Our Mission.* Retrieved January 13, 2022, from Conscious Co-Parenting Institute: https://www.conscious-coparentinginstitute.com/

Cook, J. M., Dinnen, S., Rehman, O., Bufka, L., & Courtois, C. (2011). Responses of a sample of practicing psychologists to questions about clinical work with trauma and interest in specialized training. *Psychological Trauma: Theory, Research, Practice, and Policy, 3*(3), 253-257. doi: https://doi.org/10.1037/a0025048

Cooper, K. M., Gin, L. E., & Brownell, S. E. (2020, June 4). Depression as a concealable stigmatized identity: what influences whether students conceal or reveal their depression in undergraduate research experiences? *International Journal of Stem Education, 7*(27). doi:https://doi.org/10.1186/s40594-020-00216-5

Cotter, G. (2023, January 13). (A. M.-A. Price-Tobler, Interviewer) Wollongong, NSW, Australia.

Courtois, C. A. (2004). Complex Trauma, Complex Reactions: Assessment and Treatment. *Psychotherapy: Theory, Research, Practice, Training, 41*(4), 412-425. doi:http://dx.doi.org.ezproxy.usc.edu.au:2048/10.1037/0033-3204.41.4.412

Courtois, C. A., & Ford, J. D. (2009). *Treating complex traumatic stress disorders: An evidence-based guide.* The Guildford Press.

Cresswell, J. W. (2003). *Research Design: Qualitative, Quantitative, and Mixed Methods Approaches.* SAGE Publications Ltd.

Cresswell, J. W., & Poth, C. N. (2017). *Qualitative Inquiry and Research Design. Choosing Among Five Approaches.* Thousand Oaks, California, America: Sage Publications.

Critchfield, K. L., & Benjamin, L. S. (2008). Internalized representations of early interpersonal experience and adult relationships: a test of copy process theory in clinical and non-clinical settings. *Psychiatry, Interpersonal & Biological Processes, 71*(1), 71-92. doi:10.1521/psyc.2008.71.1.71

Cromby, J. (1999). *What's wrong with social constructionism.* Leics, England, UK: Loughborough University. Retrieved April 3, 2023, from https://www.academia.edu/767706/Whats_wrong_with_social_constructionism

Darnall, D. (1998). *Divorce Casualties. Protecting your Children From Parental Alienation.* Lanham, Maryland, USA: Taylor Trade Publishing. Retrieved January 9, 2021

Darnall, D., & Steinberg, B. F. (2008). Motivational models for spontaneous reunification with. *American Journal of Family Therapy, 36*(2), 107-115. doi:https://doi.org/10.1080/01926180701643131

Das, C. (2016). *British-Indian Adult Children of Divorce* (Vol. 1). New York, NY, USA: Ashgate Publishing.

Das, C. (2016). *British-Indian Adult Children of Divorce. Context, Impact and Coping.* (2 ed.). New York, NY, USA: Routledge Publishing.

De Bellis, M. D. (2001, September 27). Developmental traumatology: The psychobiological development of maltreated children and its implications for research, treatment, and policy. *Development and Psychopathology, 13*(3), 539-564. doi: https://doi.org/10.1017/S0954579401003078

De Quervain, D., Schwabe, L., & Roozendaal, B. (2017, January). Stress, glucocorticoids and memory: implications for treating fear-related disorders. *Nature Reviews. Neuroscience, 18*(1), 7-19. doi:DOI:10.1038/nrn.2016.155

Debowska, A., Boduszek, D., & Dhingra, K. (2015, March-April). Victim, perpetrator, and offense characteristics in filicide and filicide–suicide. *Aggression and Violent Behaviour, 21*, 113-124. doi:https://doi.org/10.1016/j.avb.2015.01.011

Denzin, N. K., & Lincoln, Y. S. (2000). *Handbook of Qualitative Research* (2 ed., Vol. 2). London: SAGE publications.

Devinsky, O. (2000). Right Cerebral Hemisphere Dominance for a Sense of Corporeal and Emotional Self. *Epilepsy & Behavior, 1*(1), 60-73. doi:https://doi.org/10.1006/ebeh.2000.0025

Downey, J. C., Gudmunson, C. G., Pang, Y. C., & Lee, K. (2017, February 8). Adverse Childhood Experiences Affect Health Risk Behaviors and Chronic Health of Iowans. *Journal of Family Violence, 32*, 557-564. doi:https://doi-org.ezproxy.usc.edu.au/10.1007/s10896-017-9909-4

DuMont, K. A., Widom, C. S., & Czaja, S. J. (2007). Predictors of resilience in abused and neglected children grown-up: The role of individual and neighborhood characteristics. *Child Abuse & Neglect, 31*(3), 255-274. doi:https://doi.org/10.1016/j.chiabu.2005.11.015

Eeny Meeny Miny Mo Foundation. (n.d.). *What is Parental Alienation.* Retrieved July 30, 2021, from Eeny Meeny Miny Mo Foundation: https://emmm.org.au/parental-alienation

Egeland, B., Jacobvitz, D., & Sroufe, A. L. (1988, August 1). Breaking the cycle of abuse. *Society for Research in Child Development, 59*(4), 1080-1088. doi:10.2307/1130274

Ellis, A. E., Gold, S. N., Courtois, C., Araujo, K., & Quinones, M. (2019). Supervising Trauma Treatment: The Contextual Trauma Treatment Model Applied to Supervision. *Practice Innovations, 4*(3), 166-181. doi:https://doi.org/10.1037/pri0000095

Elshaikh, E. M. (n.d). *Standing on the Shoulders of Invisible Giants.* Retrieved August 4, 2023, from Khan Academy: https://www.khanacademy.org/humanities/big-history-project/big-bang/how-did-big-bang-change/a/standing-on-the-shoulders-of-invisible-giants

Erel, D. (2022). *Handling Parental Alienation as a Medical Emergency.* Retrieved January 13, 2022, from Parental Alienation Study Group: https://pasg.info/app/uploads/2019/07/Erel_Medical_Emergency_2019_11.pdf

Fares, R., Najem, R., Hallit, S., Pelissolo, A., Haddad, G., & Naja, W. J. (2023, April 23). Parental alienation in Lebanon: a case report. *Journal of Medical Case Reports, 17*(1), 1-12. doi:doi: 10.1186/s13256-023-03911-3

Felitti, V. J., Anda, R. F., Nordenberg, D., Williamson, D. F., Spitz, A. M., Edwards, V., . . . Marks, J. S. (1998). Relationship of Childhood Abuse and Household Dysfunction to Many of the Leading Causes of Death in Adults. *American Journal of Preventative Medicine, 14*(4), 245-258. doi:https://doi.org/10.1016/S0749-3797(98)00017-8

Fidler, B. J., & Bala, N. (2010, January 15). Children Resisting Postseparation Contact With a Parent: Concepts, Controversies, and Conundrums. *Family Court Review. An Interdisciplinary Journal, 48*(1). doi:https://doi-org.ezproxy.usc.edu.au/10.1111/j.1744-1617.2009.01287.x

Fidler, B., Bala, N., & Saini, M. (2012). *Children Who Resist PostSeparation Parental Contact: A Different Approach For Legal and Mental Health Professionals.* New York: Oxford University Press.

Fine, M., Weis, L., Weseen, S., & Wong, L. (2000). *For Whom? Qualitative research, representations, and social responsibilities.* Thousand Oaks, California, USA: Sage.

Finkelhor, D., & Browne, A. (1985). THE TRAUMATIC IMPACT OF CHILD SEXUAL ABUSE: A Conceptualization. *American Journal of Orthopsychiatry, 55*(4), 530-541. doi:http://dx.doi.org.ezproxy.usc.edu.au:2048/10.1111/j.1939-0025.1985.tb02703.x

Finlay, L. (2011). *Phenomenology for Therapists Researching the Lived World* (Vol. 1). Chichester, West Sussex, United Kingdom: John Wiley & Sons Ltd.

Flaskerud, J. H., & Winslow, B. W. (2010, March 10). Vulnerable Populations and Ultimate Responsibility. *Issues in Mental Health Nursing, 31*(4), 298-299. doi:https://doi.org/10.3109/01612840903308556

Fonagy, P., & Luyten, P. (2019, September 9). Fidelity vs. flexibility in the implementation of psychotherapies: time to move on. *World Psychiatry, 18*(3), 270-271. doi: https://doi.org/10.1002/wps.20657

Foucault, M. (1988). *Technologies of the Self.* (P. H. Hutton, H. Gutman, & L. H. Martin, Eds.) University of Vermont, Vermont, USA.

Galanena, C. (2019). Presentation-child abuse. (pp. 1-4). Campbelltown: Western Sydney University. Retrieved December 5, 2022, from https://www.studocu.com/en-au/document/western-sydney-university/child-abuse-as-a-social-issue/presentation-child-abuse/8770829

Galbin, A. (2014, December). An introduction to social constructionism. *Social Research Reports, 26*, 82-92. Retrieved March 31, 2023, from https://www.proquest.com/docview/1752382689?accountid=28745&parentSessionId=0GmTKmvk5OFYnCRHiE9IRFo1ammo4Tj6wnZQt8Qlz-t8%3D&pq-origsite=primo

Garber, B. D. (2004). Therapist Alienation: Foreseeing and Forestalling Third-Party Dynamics Undermining Psychotherapy With Children of Conflicted Caregivers. *Professional Psychology: Research and Practice, 35*(4), 357-363. doi:doi:10.1037/0735-7028.35.4.357

Gardner, R. A. (1992). The Parental Alienation Syndrome: A Guide for Mental Health and Legal Professionals-Addendum. In R. A. Gardner, *The Parental Alienation Syndrome: A Guide for Mental Health and Legal Professionals* (pp. Addendum 1-6). Cresskill, New Jersey, America: Creative Therapeutics.

Gardner, R. A. (1998, October 12). Recommendations for Dealing with Parents who Induce a Parental Alienation Syndrome in their Children. *Journal of Divorce & Remarriage, 28*(3-4), 1-23. doi:https://doi.org/10.1300/J087v28n03_01

Gardner, R. A. (1998). *The parental alienation syndrome: A guide for mental health and legal professionals* (2nd ed.). Cresskill, NJ, USA: Creative Therapeutics.

Gelinas, D. J. (1983). The persisting negative effects of incest. *Psychiatry: Journal for the Study of Interpersonal Processes, 46*(4), 312-332. Retrieved January 17, 2021, from https://psycnet.apa.org/record/1984-20729-001

Gentner, M. B., & O'Connor-Leppert, M. L. (2019). Environmental influences on health and development: nutrition, substance exposure, and adverse childhood experiences. *Developmental Medicine & Child Neurology, 61*(9), 989-1116. doi:https://doi.org/10.1111/dmcn.14149

Gerba, C. P. (2019). *Environmental and Pollution Science* (3 ed.). (M. L. Brusseau, I. L. Pepper, & C. P. Gerba, Eds.) Tucson, Arizona, America: Academic Press. doi:https://doi.org/10.1016/C2017-0-00480-9

Gerhardt, C. (2019). *Families in Motion: Dynamics in Diverse Contexts.* (S. University, Ed.) Birmingham, Alabama, USA: SAGE Publications, Inc.

Giancarlo, C. (2019). *Parentectomy.* Victoria, BC, Canada: Tell Well Talent.

Giorgi, A. (2009). *The Descriptive Phenomenological Method in Psychology: A Modified Husserlian Approach.* Duquesne University Press.

Giorgi, A. (2009). *The descriptive phenomenological method in psychology; a modified Husserlian approach.* Pittsburgh, USA: Duquesne Press.

Given, L. M. (2008). *Lived Experience* (Vols. 1-0). Thousand Oaks, California, America: The SAGE Encyclopedia of Qualitative Research Methods. doi:https://dx-doi-org.ezproxy.usc.edu.au/10.4135/9781412963909.n250

Godbout, E., & Parent, C. (2012, January 23rd). The Life Paths and Lived Experiences of Adults Who Have Experienced Parental Alienation: A Retrospective Study. *Journal of Divorce & Remarriage, 53*(1), 34-54. doi:https://doi-org.ezproxy.usc.edu.au/10.1080/10502556.2012.635967

Godin, K., Stapleton, J., Kirkpatrick, S. I., Hanning, R. M., & Leatherdale, S. T. (2015, October 22). Applying systematic review search methods to the grey literature: a case study examining guidelines for school-based breakfast programs in Canada. *Systematic Reviews, 4*(138), 27. doi:https://doi.org/10.1186/s13643-015-0125-0

Goldin, D. S., & Salani, D. (2020, May). Parental Alienation Syndrome: What Health Care Providers Need to Know. *The Journal for Nurse Practitioners, 16*(5), 344-348. doi:https://doi.org/10.1016/j.nurpra.2020.02.006

Gomez, A., Chinchilla, J., Vazquez, A., Lopez-Rodriguez, L., Paredes, B., & Martinez, M. (2020, April 23). Recent advances, misconceptions, untested assumptions, and future research agenda for identity fusion theory. *Social and Personality Psychology Compass, 14*(6), 1-24. doi:https://doi-org.ezproxy.usc.edu.au/10.1111/spc3.12531

Goodman, R. (2017). Contemporary Trauma Theory and Trauma-Informed Care in Substance Use Disorders: A Conceptual Model for Integrating Coping and Resilience. *Advances in Social Work, 18*(1), 186-201. doi:10.18060/21312

Green, J. G., McLaughlin, K. A., Berglund, P. A., Gruber, M. J., Sampson, N. A., Zaslavsky, A. M., & Kessler, R. C. (2010). Childhood adversities and adult psychiatric disorders in the National Comorbidity Survey Replication I: Associations with first onset of DSM-IV disorders. *Archives of General Psychiatry, 67*(2), 113-123. doi:https://doi-org.ezproxy.usc.edu.au/10.1001/archgenpsychiatry.2009.186

Gye, B. (2023, May 3). CEO Community Mental Health Australia. (A. M. Price-Tobler, Interviewer) NSW, Australia.

Haines, J., Matthewson, M., & Turnbull, M. (2020). *Understanding and Managing Parental Alienation. A Guide to Assessment and Intervention.* (Vol. 1). Abingdon, Oxon, England: Routledge. Retrieved October 31, 2020

Hamilton, J. C., & Kouchi, K. A. (2018, January 5). Factitious Disorders and the Adjudication of Claims of Physical and Mental Injury. *Psychological Injury and Law*(N/A), 9-21. doi:https://doi-org.ezproxy.usc.edu.au/10.1007/s12207-017-9310-x

Harman, J. (2016). 'Parental alienation': What it means and why it matters. *The Conversation*, 1-5. Retrieved January 16, 2021, from https://theconversation.com/parental-alienation-what-it-means-and-why-it-matters-60763

Harman, J. J., Leder-Elder, S., & Biringen, Z. (2019). Prevalence of adults who are the targets of parental alienating behaviors and their impact. *Children and Youth Services Review, 106*, 1-21. doi:doi.org/10.1016/j.childyouth.2019.104471

Harman, J. J., Matthewson, M. L., & Baker, A. J. (2021, May 10). Losses Experienced by Children Alienated from a Parent. *Current Opinion in Psychology*, 1-21. doi:https://doi.org/10.1016/j.copsyc.2021.05.002

Harper, D. (2008). *Reflexivity: A Practical Guide for Researchers in Health and Social Sciences.* Oxford.

Harris, C. H. (2008). Intimate partner homicide and familicide in Western Australia. *International conference on homicide.* Retrieved May 28, 2023, from https://usc.primo.exlibrisgroup.com/discovery/fulldisplay?docid=cdi_rmit_indexes_9781921532429er_homicide_and_familicide_in_Western_Au_62207_CINCH_Health&context=PC&vid=61USC_INST:61USC&lang=en&search_scope=CentralIndex&adaptor=Primo%20Central&tab=Central

Henderson, A. (2018). *Enid Lyons. Leading Lady to a Nation* (2 ed.). Redlands Bay, Qld, Australia: Jeparit Press.

Herman, J. (1992). Complex PTSD: A syndrome in survivors of prolonged and repeated trauma. *Journal of Traumatic Stress, 5*(3), 377-391. doi:10.1002/jts.2490050305

Herman, J. L. (2002, January 4). Recovery from psychological trauma. *Psychiatry and Clinical Neurosciences, 52*(1), S98-S103. doi:https://doi-org.ezproxy.usc.edu.au/10.1046/j.1440-1819.1998.0520s5S145.x

Hertz, R. (1997). *Reflexivity and Voice.* SAGE Publications Inc.

Hesse-Bibber, S. N., & Piatelli, D. (2012). *The Feminist Practice of Holistic Reflexivity.* Sage Publications Inc. doi:https://doi.org/10.4135/9781483384740

Hetherington, M. E. (1993). An overview of the Virginia Longitudinal Study of Divorce and Remarriage with a focus on early adolescence. *Journal of Family Psychology, 7*(1), 39-56. doi:http://dx.doi.org.ezproxy.usc.edu.au:2048/10.1037/0893-3200.7.1.39

Hickey, S., & Nedim, U. (2020, August 25). *Abducting Your Own Child Can Amount to a Crime in Australia.* Retrieved June 19, 2021, from Sydney Criminal Lawyers: https://www.mondaq.com/australia/crime/979016/abducting-your-own-child-can-amount-to-a-crime-in-australia

Horsfall, D., & Pinn, J. (2009). Writing collaboratively. In S. Grace (Ed.). The Netherlands: Sense Publishers. Retrieved November 5, 2022, from https://researchdirect.westernsydney.edu.au/islandora/object/uws%3A25977

Hughes, A. E., Crowell, S. E., Uyeji, L., & Coan, J. A. (2012, January). A Developmental Neuroscience of Borderline Pathology: Emotion

Dysregulation and Social Baseline Theory. *Journal of Abnormal Child Psychology, 40*(1), 21-33. doi:10.1007/s10802-011-9555-x

ISNAF. (2021). *Parental Alienation Glossary of Terms.* Retrieved January 16, 2021, from The International Support Network of Alienated Families: https://isnaf.info/parental-alienation-glossary-of-terms/

Jaber, N. (2021, January 14). *NIH National Cancer Institute.* Retrieved June 30, 2023, from Study Suggests a Link Between Stress and Cancer Coming Back: https://www.cancer.gov/news-events/cancer-currents-blog/2021/cancer-returning-stress-hormones

Jaffe, P. G., Campbell, M., Hamilton, L. H., & Juodis, M. (2012). Children in Danger of Domestic Homicide. *Chile Abuse & Neglect, 36*(1), 71-74. doi:doi: 10.1016/j.chiabu.2011.06.008

Jaffe, P., Dawson, M., & Campbell, M. (2013). Canadian perspectives on preventing domestic homicides: Developing a national collaborative approach to domestic homicide review committees. *Canadian Journal of Criminology and Criminal Justice Policy, 55*(1), 137-155. doi:Doi: 10.3138/cjccj.2011.E.53

Johnson, C. H. (2005). *Come with Daddy: Child Murder-Suicide After Family Breakdown.* Crawley, W.A: The University of Western Australia Publishing. doi:DOI: 10.3316/informit.1920694420

Johnson, C. H. (2008). Intimate partner homicide and familicide in Western Australia. *International conference on homicide.* Australian Criminology Database. Retrieved May 28, 2023, from https://usc.primo.exlibrisgroup.com/discovery/fulldisplay?docid=cdi_rmit_indexes_9781921532429er_homicide_and_familicide_in_Western_Au_62207_CINCH_Health&context=PC&vid=61USC_INST:61USC&lang=en&search_scope=CentralIndex&adaptor=Primo%20Central&tab=Central

Johnson, C. H. (2009). "Intimate Partner Homicide, Familicide and Child Trauma and the Need for. (pp. 1-9). Curtin University of Technology. Retrieved May 28, 2023, from https://aija.org.au/wp-content/uploads/2017/11/Johnson1.pdf

Jones, E. (1991). *Working with Adult Survivors of Child Sexual Abuse.* London, England: Routledge.

Judd, F., Jackson, H., Fraser, C., Murray, G., Robins, G., & Komiti, A. (2006). Understanding suicide in Australian farmers. *Social Psychiatry and*

Psychiatric Epidemiology, 41(1), 1-10. doi:https://doi.org/10.1007/s00127-005-0007-1

Karlsson, L. C., Antfolk, J., Putkonen, H., Amon, S., Guerreiro, J. d., De Vogel, V., . . . Weizmann-Henelius, G. (2021). Familicide: A Systematic Literature Review. *TRAUMA, VIOLENCE, & ABUSE, 22*(1), 83-98. doi:https://doi.org/10.1177/1524838018821955

Kelly, J. B. (2010). Commentary on "family bridges: using insights from social science to reconnect parents and alienation children" (Warshak, 2010). *Family Court Review, 48*(1), 81-90. doi:https://doi.org/10.1111/j.1744-1617.2009.01289.x

Kessler, R. R. (2000). Posttraumatic stress disorder: The burden to the individual and to society. *The Journal of Clinical Psychiatry, 61*(5), 4-14. Retrieved August 28, 2021, from https://psycnet-apa-org.ezproxy.usc.edu.au/record/2000-15312-001

Kilpatrick, D. G., Ruggiero, K. J., Acierno, R., Saunders, B. E., Resnick, H. S., & Best, C. (2003). Violence and risk of PTSD, major depression, substance abuse/dependence, and comorbidity: Results from the National Survey of Adolescents. *Journal of Consulting and Clinical Psychology, 71*(4), 692-700. doi:https://doi.org/10.1037/0022-006X.71.4.692

King, N. (2004). *Using Interviews in Qualitative Research.* London: SAGE Publications Ltd.

Kirkwood, D. (2012). *'Just say goodbye': parents who kill their children in the context of separation.* Discussion paper, Domestic Violence Resource Centre, Victoria, Collingwood. Retrieved May 28, 2023, from https://vgls.sdp.sirsidynix.net.au/client/search/asset/1288903

Kleinsorge, C., & Covitz, L. M. (2012, April). Impact of Divorce on Children: Developmental Considerations. *Pediatrics in Review*, 147-155. doi:https://doi.org/10.1542/pir.33-4-147

Korosi, S. (2017, November 4). *Overcoming Parental Alienation.* Retrieved January 11, 2022, from Dialogue in Growth: https://dialogueingrowth.com.au/parental-alienationevidence-based-reunification-available-in-australia/

Kotze, D. (2020, January 30). FW de Klerk made a speech 31 years ago that ended apartheid: why he did it. *The Conversation*, 1-4. Retrieved December 4, 2022, from https://theconversation.com/fw-de-klerk-made-a-speech-31-years-ago-that-ended-apartheid-why-he-did-it-130803

Kruk, E. (2022). *Strategies to reunite alienated parents and their children.* Retrieved January 11, 2022, from Child Rights NGO: https://childrightsngo.com/parent-child-reunification-after-alienation/

Larsson, S. C., Carter, P., Kar, S., Vithayathil, M., Mason, A. M., Michaelsson, K., & Burgess, S. (2020, July 23). Smoking, alcohol consumption, and cancer: A mendelian randomisation study in UK Biobank and international genetic consortia participants. *PLoS Medicine, 17*(7). doi:doi: 10.1371/journal.pmed.1003178

Lauterbach, A. A. (2018, November). Hermeneutic Phenomenological Interviewing: Going Beyond Semi-Structured Formats to Help Participants Revisit Experience. *The Qualitative Report, 23*(11), 2882-2898. Retrieved July 10, 2021, from https://www-proquest-com.ezproxy.usc.edu.au/docview/2155621343?pq-origsite=primo&accountid=28745

Lee-Maturana, S., Matthewson, M. L., & Dwan, C. (2020, May 18). Targeted Parents Surviving Parental Alienation: Consequences of the Alienation and Coping Strategies. *Journal of Child and Family Studies, 29*, 1-49. doi:https://doi-org.ezproxy.usc.edu.au/10.1007/s10826-020-01725-1

Lewis, C. F., & Bunce, S. C. (2003, December). Filicidal mothers and the impact of psychosis on maternal filicide. *The Journal of the American Academy of Psychiatry and the Law, 31*(4), 459-470. Retrieved 28 5, 2023, from https://jaapl.org/content/31/4/459

Lewis, D. (2003). Voices in the social construction of bullying at work: exploring multiple realities in further and higher education. *International Journal of Decision Making, 4*(1), 65-81. Retrieved December 5, 2022, from https://www.researchgate.net/publication/247831471_Voices_in_the_social_construction_of_bullying_at_work_exploring_multiple_realities_in_further_and_higher_education

Liamputtong, P. (2019). *Sensitive Research Methodology and Approach: An Introduction.* Singapore: Springer Nature. doi:https://doi.org/10.1007/978-981-10-5251-4_122

Liebrucks, A. (2001, June). The Concept of Social Construction. *Theoretical psychology, 11*(3), 363-391. doi:https://doi-org.ezproxy.usc.edu.au/10.1177/0959354301113005

Linabary, J. R., Corple, D. J., & Cooky, C. (2020, August 29). Of wine and whiteboards: Enacting feminist reflexivity in collaborative research.

Qualitative Research, 21(5), 719-735. doi:https://doi-org.ezproxy.usc.edu.au/10.1177/1468794120946988

Liu, S., Yang, H., Cheng, M., & Miao, T. (2022, August 7). Family Dysfunction and Cyberchondria among Chinese Adolescents: A Moderated Mediation Model. *International Journal of Environmental Research and Public Health, 19*(15), 1-23. doi: doi: 10.3390/ijerph19159716

Lo, I. (2019, December 12). *Did You Have to Grow Up Too Soon?* Retrieved June 16, 2021, from Psychology Today: https://www.psychologytoday.com/au/blog/living-emotional-intensity/201912/did-you-have-grow-too-soon

Locke, E. (2001). Motivation, Cognition, and Action: An Analysis of Studies of Task Goals and Knowledge. *Applied Psychology, 49*(3), 408-429. doi: https://doi-org.ezproxy.usc.edu.au/10.1111/1464-0597.00023

Lorandos, D., & Bernet, W. (2020). *Parental Alienation Science and Law.* Springfield, Illinois, America: Charles C Thomas. Retrieved November 6, 2020

Lorandos, D., Bernet, W., & Sauber, S. R. (2013). *Overview of Parental Alienation, in Parental Alienation: The Handbook for Mental Health and Legal Professionals.* (B. a. Lorandos, Ed.) Springfield, Illinois, America: Charles C Thomas.

Mahmood, K. (2006). Dr. Elisabeth Kubler-Ross stages of dying and phenomenology of grief. *Annals of King Edward Medical University, 12*(2), 232-233. doi:DOI: https://doi.org/10.21649/akemu.v12i2.882

Martin, J., & Pritchard, R. (2010). *Learning from tragedy : homicide within families in New Zealand 2002-2006.* Retrieved May 28 2023, from New Zealand Family Violence Clearinghouse: https://library.nzfvc.org.nz/cgi-bin/koha/opac-detail.pl?biblionumber=2490

McCann, L. I., & Pearlman, L. A. (1990, August 28). Vicarious traumatization: A framework for understanding the psychological effects of working with victims. *Journal of Traumatic Stress, 3*(1), 131-149. Retrieved August 28, 2021, from https://psycnet-apa-org.ezproxy.usc.edu.au/record/1990-17844-001

McCarty, D. E. (2020, March 22). Parental Alienation: Eric Carroll--Dad Talk Today host--flips the questions back to Dawn and Alyse. *Dad Talk Today.* (E. Carroll, Interviewer, & A. Price-Tobler, Editor) Florida, America. Retrieved June 7, 7.6.2021, from https://humanlypossiblechannel.com/humanly-possible-videos

McGowan, A. (2021, July 24). Radicalism mixed with openness: how Desmond Tutu used his gifts to help end Apartheid. *The Conversation*, 1-5. Retrieved December 4, 2022, from https://theconversation.com/radicalism-mixed-with-openness-how-desmond-tutu-used-his-gifts-to-help-end-apartheid-156499

McLaughlin, K. A., Green, J. G., Berglund, P. A., Gruber, M. J., Sampson, N. A., Zaslavsky, A. M., & Kessler, R. C. (2010). Childhood adversities and adult psychiatric disorders in the National Comorbidity Survey Replication I: Associations with first onset of DSM-IV disorders. *Archives of General Psychiatry, 67*(2), 113-123. doi: https://doi-org.ezproxy.usc.edu.au/10.1001/archgenpsychiatry.2009.186

McWhorter, M. R. (2019, August 13). Balancing Value Bracketing with the Integration of Moral Values in Psychotherapy: Evaluation of a Clinical Practice from the Perspective of Catholic Moral Theology. *The Linacre Quarterly, 86*(2-3), 207-224. doi:doi: 10.1177/0024363919856810

Mead, G. H. (1934). *MIND, SELF, and SOCIETY from the standpoint of a social behaviorist.* Chicago, United States: The University of Chicago Press.

Meland, E., Furuholmen, D., & Jahanlu, D. (2023, April 23). Parental alienation – a valid experience? *Scandinavian Journal of Public Health, 0*(0), 1-14. doi:https://doi.org/10.1177/14034948231168978

Merriam, S. B., & Tisdell, E. J. (2016). *Qualitative research: A guide to design and implementation* (4 ed.). San Francisco, America: Newark-Wiley.

Metzler, M., Merrick, M. T., Klevens, J., Ports, K. A., & Ford, D. C. (2017). Adverse childhood experiences and life opportunities: Shifting the narrative. *Children and Youth Services Review, 72*, 141-149. doi:https://doi.org/10.1016/j.childyouth.2016.10.021

Michalchuk, S., & Martin, S. L. (2019). Vicarious Resilience and Growth in Psychologists Who Work With Trauma Survivors: An Interpretive Phenomenological Analysis. *Professional Psychology: Research and Practice, 50*(3), 145-154. doi:http://dx.doi.org.ezproxy.usc.edu.au:2048/10.1037/pro0000212

Milloy, J. (2010). Attending to the somatic fringes of the moment (panel presentation). *International Human Science Research Conference.* Seattle.

Montagna, P. (2019). Parental alienation and parental alienation syndrome. In *Psychoanalysis, Law, and Society* (pp. 188-200). Routledge. doi:10.4324/9780429202438

Moon, K., & Blackman, D. (2017, May 2). *A guide to ontology, epistemology, and philosophical perspectives for interdisciplinary researchers.* Retrieved May 13, 2023, from Integration and Implementation Insights: https://i2insights.org/2017/05/02/philosophy-for-interdisciplinarity/#:~:text=and%20Blackman%202014)-,Ontology,of%20objects%20they%20are%20researching.

Morgan, A., Ahmad, N., & Webster, M. (2020). *The Clinical and Legal Management of Parental Alienation in the United Kingdom.* Final Report, University of Wolver Hampton. Retrieved January 13, 2022, from https://pasg.info/app/uploads/2021/03/Morgan-et-al.-2020-PA-in-UK.pdf

Mouzos, J., & Rushforth, C. (2003). Family homicide in Australia. *Trends & issues in Crime and Criminal Justice*(255), 1-6. Retrieved May 28, 2023, from https://www.aic.gov.au/publications/tandi/tandi255

Muris, P., Merckelbach, H., de Jong, P. J., & Ollendick, T. H. (2002, February). The etiology of specific fears and phobias in children: a critique of the non-associative account. *Behaviour Research and Therapy, 40*(2), 185-195. doi:https://doi.org/10.1016/S0005-7967(01)00051-1

National Library of Medicine. (2003). Chapter 3 The Core Competencies Needed for Health Care Professionals. In *Health Professions Education* (pp. 1-25). Bethesda, MD, USA. Retrieved December 4, 2022, from https://www.ncbi.nlm.nih.gov/books/NBK221519/

National School of Healthcare Science. (n.d.). *Understanding different types of bias*. Retrieved May 14, 2023, from NHS England: https://nshcs.hee.nhs.uk/about/equality-diversity-and-inclusion/conscious-inclusion/understanding-different-types-of-bias/

Natoli, A. P., Paez, M. M., & McGowan, T. (2022, June 17). Psychodynamic psychotherapy. *Reference Module in Neuroscience and Biobehavioural Psychology.* doi:https://doi.org/10.1016/B978-0-323-91497-0.00074-6

Nesvig, K. (2022, February 3). *The Simple, 5-Minute Habits That Therapists Say Will Reduce WFH Burnout.* Retrieved December 5, 2022, from Apartment Therapy: https://www.apartmenttherapy.com/habits-reduce-work-from-home-burnout-37032803

Newby, J. M., & McElroy, E. (2020, January). The impact of internet-delivered cognitive behavioural therapy for health anxiety on cyberchondria. *Journal of Anxiety Disorders, 69*, 1-8. doi:https://doi.org/10.1016/j.janxdis.2019.102150

Nowell, L. S., Norris, J. M., White, D. E., & Moules, N. J. (2017, October 2). Thematic Analysis: Striving to Meet the Trustworthiness Criteria. *International Journal of Qualitative Methods, 16*(1), 1-13. doi:10.1177/1609406917733847

NSW Government Health. (2020, January 20). *What is a person-centred approach?* Retrieved February 16, 2021, from NSW Government Health: https://www.health.nsw.gov.au/mentalhealth/psychosocial/principles/Pages/person-centred.aspx

Office of Juvenile Justice and Delinquency Prevention. (2010). *The Crime of Family Abduction. A Child's and Parent's Perspective.* Washington , D.C, America: U.S Department of Justice. Retrieved June 19, 2021, from https://www.ojp.gov/pdffiles1/ojjdp/229933.pdf?fbclid=IwAR3l-r7mcC6eC3vCgzpT6Z8rbt70i9r7ou0pSZJHMBkopGP6cs9UgLyKfuL0

One Door Mental Health. (2020, June). *Join Our Board.* Retrieved August 17, 2023, from One Door Mental Health: https://www.onedoor.org.au/news-updates/enews/enews-june-2020/join-our-board

Opperman, J. (2004, July-August). Parental Alienation Syndrome: what do you do when your child stops seeing you as mom or dad? *Children's Voice, 13*(4), 23-25. Retrieved August 14, 2021, from https://www-proquest-com.ezproxy.usc.edu.au/docview/203947284?accountid=28745

Pang, B. (2019). *Handbook of Research Methods in Health Social Sciences Ethnographic Method.* (P. Liamputtong, Ed.) Singapore: Springer Nature. doi:https://doi.org/10.1007/978-981-10-5251-4_81

Parental Alienation Study Group. (2022). *PASG info.* Retrieved February 28, 2022, from Parental Alienation Study Group: https://pasg.info/

Peavey, F. (1990). *Strategic Questioning Manual: A Powerful Tool for Personal and Social Change.* Retrieved July 10, 2021, from The Commons Social Change Library: https://commonslibrary.org/strategic-questioning/

Perry, B. D. (2003). *Effects of Traumatic Events on Children.* Retrieved July 20, 2021, from Child Trauma Academy. A Learning Community: http://fa-sett.no/filer/perry-handout-effects-of-trauma.pdf

Perry, B. D. (2021). *ChildTrauma Academy History.* Retrieved July 20, 2021, from ChildTrauma Academy: https://7079168e-705a-4dc7-be05-2218087aa989.filesusr.com/ugd/aa51c7_237459a7e16b4b7e9d2c4837c908eefe.pdf

Peterson, A. J., Joseph, J., Feit, M., Medicine, I., & Council, N. (2014). *New Directions in Child Abuse and Neglect Research.* National Academies Press. doi:DOI:10.17226/18331

Pham, M. T., Rajic, A., Greig, J. D., Sargeant, J. M., Papadopoulos, A., & McEwen, S. A. (2014, July 24). Wiley Research Synthesis Methods. *PMC US National Library of Medicine National Institutes of Health, 5*(4), 371-385. doi:10.1002/jrsm.1123

Pier, K. S., Marin, L. K., Wilsnack, J., & Goodman, M. (2016, April 1). The Neurobiology of Borderline Personality Disorder. *Psychiatric Times, 33*(3), 1-7. Retrieved June 7, 2021, from Psychiatric Times: https://www.psychiatrictimes.com/view/neurobiology-borderline-personality-disorder

Price-Tobler, A. M. (2023). *https://www.alyseprice-tobler.com/specialities.* Retrieved from https://www.alyseprice-tobler.com/: https://www.alyse-price-tobler.com/

Putkonen, H., Eronon, M., Almiron, M., Cederwall, J., & Weizmann-Henelius, G. (2011). Gender Differences in Filicide Offense Characteristics-A Comprehensive Register Based Study of Child Murder in Two European Countries. *Child abuse and neglect, 35*(5), 319-328. doi:doi: 10.1016/j.chiabu.2011.01.007

Raheim, M., Magnussen, L. H., Sekse, R. J., Lunde, A., Jacobsen, T., & Blystad, A. (2016, June 14). Researcher–researched relationship in qualitative research: Shifts in positions and researcher vulnerability. *International Journal of Qualitative Studies in Health and Well-being, 11.* doi:doi: 10.3402/qhw.v11.30996

Rand, D. C. (1997, December 16). The Spectrum of Parental Alienation Syndrome (PART II). *American Journal of Forensic Psychology, 15*(4), 1. Retrieved March 20, 2020, from https://canadiancrc.com/Parental_Alienation_Syndrome_Canada/randp2.pdf

Reinharz, S. (1992). *Feminist methods in social research.* New York: Oxford University Press.

Resnick, P. J. (1969, September). Child Murder by Parents: A Psychiatric Review of Filicide. *The American Journal of Psychiatry, 126*(3), 352-334. doi:https://doi.org/10.1176/ajp.126.3.325

Roberts, R. (2020, June 6). Humanly Possible Channel. (D. McCarty, & A. M. Price-Tobler, Interviewers) Retrieved June 10, 2021, from https://www.youtube.com/watch?v=CX7cBkAbzgU

Rosenberg, M. B. (2015). *Nonviolent Communication: A Language of Life* (3 ed.). (L. Leu, Ed.) Encinitas, California, USA: PuddleDancer Press.

Ross, C. A. (1989). *Multiple Personality Disorder: Diagnosis, Clinicla Features, and Treatment* (Vol. 4). Washington, DC, USA: American Psychiatric Publishing.

Ross, D. (2020). *The Revolutionary Social Worker. The Love Ethic Model.* Brisbane, Australia: Revolutionaries.

Ruggles, S. (1994, February). The Origins of African-American Family Structure. *American Sociological Review, 59*(1), 1-17. doi:10.2307/2096137

Saini, S. M., Hoffman, C. R., Pantelis, C., Everall, I. P., & Bousman, C. A. (2019, February). Systematic review and critical appraisal of child abuse measurement instruments. *Psychiatry Research, 272*, 106-113. doi:10.1016/j.psychres.2018.12.068

Salkind, N. (1991). *Exploring research* (3 ed.). (P. Janzow, Ed.) New Jersey: Simon & Schuster. Retrieved June 28, 2016

Saunders, B., Sim, J., Kingstone, T., Baker, S., Waterfield, J., Bartlam, B., . . . Jinks, C. (2017, September 14). Saturation in qualitative research: exploring its conceptualization and operationalization. *Quality and Quantity, 52*(4), 1893-1907. doi:doi: 10.1007/s11135-017-0574-8

Schore, A. N. (2002). Dysregulation of the right brain: a fundamental mechanism of traumatic attachment and the psychopathogenesis of post-traumatic stress disorder. *Australian and New Zealand Journal of Psychiatry, 36*(1), 9-30. doi:10.1046/j.1440-1614.2002.00996.x.

Schore, A. N. (2009, April 1). *Relational Trauma and the Developing Right Brain. An Interface of Psychoanalytic Self Psychology and Neuroscience.* doi:10.1111/j.1749-6632.2009.04474.x

Schultheiss, D. E., & Wallace, E. (2012). *An introduction to social constructionism in vocational psychology and career development* (Vol. 4). Brill. Retrieved March 31, 2023, from https://ebookcentral.proquest.com/lib/usc/detail.action?docID=3034785#

Scott, P. D. (1973, April). Parents who kill their Children. *HeinOnline, 13*(2), 120-126. Retrieved May 28, 2023, from https://heinonline-org.ezproxy.usc.edu.au/HOL/Page?collection=journals&handle=hein.journals/mdsclw13&id=125&men_tab=srchresults

Sher, L. (2017). Parental alienation: the impact on men's mental health. *International Journal of Adolescent Medicine and Health; Berlin, 29*(3), 1-5. doi:10.1515/ijamh-2015-0083

Shivayogi, P. (2013). Vulnerable population and methods for their safeguard. *Perspectives in Clinical Research, 4*(1), 53-57. doi:10.4103/2229-3485.106389

Silva, E., Till, A., & Adshead, G. (2018, January 2). Ethical dilemmas in psychiatry: When teams disagree. *Cambridge University Press, 23*(4), 231-239. doi:10.1192/apt.bp.116.016147

Silverman, D. (1997). *Validity and credibility in qualitative research. The alternative paradigm.* (G. Miller, & R. Dingwall, Eds.) London: Sage.

Sorsoli, L., Kia-Keating, M., Grossman, F. K., & Mallinckrodt, B. (2008). "I Keep That Hush-Hush": Male Survivors of Sexual Abuse and the Challenges of Disclosure. *Journal of counselling psychology, 55*(3), 333-345. doi:10.1037/0022-0167.55.3.333

Starcevic, V. (2017, May). Cyberchondria: Challenges of Problematic Online Searches for Health-Related Information. *Psychotherapy and Psychosomatics, 86*(3), 129-133. doi:https://doi.org/10.1159/000465525

Strang, H. (1996, March 1). *Children as victims of homicide.* Retrieved May 28, 2023, from Australian Government. Australian Institute of Criminology: https://www.aic.gov.au/publications/tandi/tandi53

Stroud, J. (2008, November 1). A psychosocial analysis of child homicide. *Critical Social Policy, 28*(4), 482-505. doi:https://doi-org.ezproxy.usc.edu.au/10.1177/0261018308095281

Sullivan, M. J., Ward, P. A., & Deutsch, R. M. (2010, January). OVERCOMING BARRIERS FAMILY CAMP: A PROGRAM FOR HIGH-CONFLICT DIVORCED FAMILIES WHERE A CHILD1 IS RESISTING CONTACT WITH A PARENT. *Family Court Review, 48*(1), 116-135. doi:10.1111/j.1744-1617.2009.01293.x

Teicher, M. H., & Samson, J. A. (2013, October 1). Childhood Maltreatment and Psychopathology: A Case for Ecophenotypic Variants as Clinically and Neurobiologically Distinct Subtypes. *The American Journal of Psychiatry.* doi:10.1176/appi.ajp.2013.12070957

Templer, K., Matthewson, M., Haines, J., & Cox, G. (2016, October 3). Recommendations for best practice in response to parental alienation:

findings from a systematic review. *Journal of Family Therapy, 39*(1), 103-122. doi:10.1111/1467-6427.12137

The ATLEN. (2017, November 26). *Aotearoa Therapists with Lived Experience Network*. Retrieved November 14, 2022, from The ATLEN: https://the-atlen.wordpress.com/2017/11/26/therapist-with-lived-experience/

Thomas, J. R., & Hognas, R. S. (2015). The Effect of Parental Divorce on the Health of Adult Children. *Longitudinal and Life Course Studies, 6*(3), 279-302. doi:10.14301/llcs.v6i3.267

Time to Put Kids First. (2019). *Home*. Retrieved 2021, from https://www.time-toputkidsfirst.org/: https://www.timetoputkidsfirst.org/

Turkat, I. D. (2000, July-September). Custody Battle Burnout. *American Journal of Family Therapy, 28*(3), 201-215. doi:10.1080/01926180050081649

University of the Health Sciences. (2021). *The Impact of Kidnapping, Shooting and Torture on Children.* Retrieved June 22, 2021, from The Center for the Study of Traumatic Stress (CSTS): https://www.cstson-line.org/resources/resource-master-list/the-impact-of-kidnapping-shooting-and-torture-on-children

van der Kolk, B. (2014). *The Body Keeps The Score* (Vol. 1). USA: Viking Penguin. Retrieved January 9 2023

van der Kolk, B. A., & Kadish, W. (1987). *Amnesia, dissociation, and the return of the repressed.* Washington, DC, USA: American Psychiatric Press.

Van Hoy, A., & Rzeszutek, M. (2022, August 15). Burnout and Psychological Wellbeing Among Psychotherapists: A Systematic Review. *Frontiers in Psychology*, 1-33. doi:10.3389/fpsyg.2022.928191

van Manen, M. (1990). *Researching Lived Experience : Human Science for an Action Sensitive Pedagogy.* Albany, New York, USA: State University of New York Press.

Verrocchio, M. C., Baker, A. J., & Bernet, W. (2016, February 16). Associations between Exposure to Alienating Behaviors, Anxiety, and Depression in an Italian Sample of Adults. *Journal of Forensic Sciences, 61*(3), 692-698. doi:10.1111/1556-4029.13046

Verrocchio, M. C., Marchetti, D., Carrozzino, D., Compare, D., & Fulcheri, M. (2019). Depression and quality of life in adults perceiving exposure to parental alienation behaviors. *Health and Quality of Life Outcomes, 17*(14), 1-9. doi:10.1186/s12955-019-1080-6

Viljoen, M., & van Rensburg, E. (2014, May 8). Exploring the Lived Experiences of Psychologists Working With Parental Alienation Syndrome. *Journal of Divorce & Remarriage, 55*(4), 253-275. doi:10.1080/10502556.2014.901833

Wallerstein, J. S. (1985). Children of Divorce: Preliminary Report of a Ten-Year Follow-up of Older Children and Adolescents. *Journal of the American Academy of Child Psychiatry, 24*(5), 545-553. doi:10.1016/S0002-7138(09)60055-8

Walter, M. (2019). *Social Research Methods* (4 ed.). (C. Leslie, Ed.) Docklands, Victoria, Australia: Oxford University Press.

Wamsley, L. (2021, June 2). *A Guide To Gender Identity Terms*. Retrieved November 19, 2022, from National Public Radio: https://www.npr.org/2021/06/02/996319297/gender-identity-pronouns-expression-guide-lgbtq#gender

Warshak, R. A. (2013). *What is Parental Alienation*. Retrieved June 26, 2021, from Dr Richard A Warshak: https://www.warshak.com/publications/what-is-parental-alienation.html

Wilcox, W. B. (2009). The Evolution of Divorce. *National Affairs*, 1-23. Retrieved July 26, 2021, from https://www.nationalaffairs.com/publications/detail/the-evolution-of-divorce#:~:text=In%201969%2C%20Governor%20Ronald,first%20no%2Dfault%20divorce%20bill.

Wilkinson, S. (1988). The role of reflexivity in feminist psychology. *Women's Studies International Forum, 11*(5), 493-502. doi:https://doi.org/10.1016/0277-5395(88)90024-6

Willig, C. (2001). *Introducing Qualitative Research in Psychology: Adventures in Theory and Method, Volume 2*. Open University Press.

Wilson, J. P., & Thomas, R. B. (2004). Empathy in the Treatment of Trauma and PTSD. Taylor & Francis Group. Retrieved February 11, 2023, from https://ebookcentral.proquest.com/lib/usc/detail.action?docID=214864&pq-origsite=primo#

Wurtz, E. T., Hansen, J., Roe, O. D., & Omland, O. (2020, February 10). Asbestos exposure and haematological malignancies: a Danish cohort study. *European Journal of Epidemiology, 35*(10), 949-960. doi:doi:10.1007/s10654-020-00609-4

Young, D. C. (2009, February). Interpretivism and Education Law Research: A Natural Fit. *Education & Law Journal, 18*(3), 203-219. Retrieved

March 12, 2023, from https://www.proquest.com/scholarly-journals/interpretivism-education-law-research-natural-fit/docview/212959444/se-2

Zachariadou, T., Zannetos, S., Chira, S. E., Gregoriou, S., & Pavlakis, A. (2018, September 7). Prevalence and Forms of Workplace Bullying Among Health-care Professionals in Cyprus: Greek Version of "Leymann Inventory of Psychological Terror" Instrument. *Science Direct, 9*(3), 339-346. doi:10.1016/j.shaw.2017.11.003

Zareen, Z., & Larsen, D. (2018, November). Commentary: Paradigms, Axiology, and Praxeology in Medical Education Research. *Academic Medicine. Journal of the Association of American Medical Colleges, 93*(11S), S1-S7. doi:10.1097/ACM.0000000000002384

A final note about references: Including all 35 pages of references in both volumes of the twin study PhD books is a strategic decision that benefits mental health practitioners and other researchers in several ways. Firstly, it provides readers with a comprehensive resource, eliminating the need to flip back and forth between volumes to access the reference list. This saves time and makes it easier for readers to locate specific sources. Additionally, having all references readily available enhances accessibility. It allows readers to cross-reference or delve deeper into specific topics covered in each volume without needing to search for the cited literature elsewhere.

Moreover, maintaining consistency across both volumes ensures the continuity of the research findings and conclusions. For researchers and academics, having access to the full list of references facilitates the verification of information, fostering trust and confidence in the research. Lastly, leaving the references intact in both volumes preserves the coherence and integrity of the content, as removing them from one of the books might disrupt the flow. Overall, this approach is a practical and valuable resource, enhancing the accessibility, credibility, and continuity of the research presented in twin study PhD books and post-doctoral research.

Appendices

✧

Appendix One

ACE Study Questions

Note: These questions were not offered to any study participants. The questions are only here for a guide to read when the study refers to 'The Ace Study'. The grammar in their list has not been corrected either.

1. Before your 18th birthday, did a parent or other adult in the household often or very often swear at you, insult you, put you down, or humiliate you? or Act in a way that made you afraid that you might be physically hurt?
2. Before your 18th birthday, did a parent or other adult in the household often or very often push, grab, slap, or throw something at you? or ever hit you so hard that you had marks or were injured?
3. Before your 18th birthday, did an adult or person at least five years older than you ever touch or fondle you or have you touched their body in a sexual way? Or Attempt or actually have oral, anal, or vaginal intercourse with you?
4. Did you often or very often feel that no one in your family loved you or thought you were important or special? Or Your family didn't look out for each other, feel close to each other, or support each other?

5. Did you often or very often feel that you didn't have enough to eat, had to wear dirty clothes, and had no one to protect you? Or Your parents were too drunk or high to take care of you or take you to the doctor if you needed it?
6. Were your parents ever separated or divorced?
7. Was your mother or stepmother often or very often pushed, grabbed, slapped, or had something thrown at her? or sometimes, often, or very often kicked, bitten, hit with a fist, or hit with something hard? or ever repeatedly hit over at least a few minutes or threatened with a gun or knife?
8. Did you live with anyone who was a problem drinker or alcoholic or who used street drugs?
9. Was a household member depressed or mentally ill, or did a household member attempt suicide?
10. Did a household member go to prison? (ACES Too High News, 2020, p. 1)

https://form.jotform.com/221574555560054

Appendix Two

Qualifying Questions for Adult Survivors of SPA

1. *Were you alienated from a parent when you were a child?*
2. *Do you identify as having one of your parents turn you against your other parent as a child?*
3. *Have you reunited with your alienated parent?*
4. *Do you identify as belonging to the 'severe' parental alienation category instead of mild or moderate?*
5. *Were you under the age of 8 when your parents divorced?*
6. *Have you had therapy from a mental health practitioner to understand more about your alienation experience?*
7. *If so, what worked, what did not and why?*

These studies looked at the perspectives of adult survivors who identify as belonging to the 'severe' category of parental alienation. Adult survivors of SPA must have received treatment as an adult for severe parental alienation from a mental health practitioner.

Appendix Three

Categories of Parental Alienation- Mild, Moderate and Severe

Please read over the following definitions of parental alienation and see which one you identify with the most. The study is looking to recruit adult-child survivors of severe parental alienation. If you feel after reading these definitions that you relate to the severe category of parental alienation, please contact Alyse Price-Tobler to apply to be in the main study.

Mild Parental Alienation

The mild type of PAS behaviour has some degree of parental programming aimed against the TP; however, visits are not detrimentally affected, and the child can manage the transition to being around the alienated TP without too much stress (Baker, 2007). A mild level of PA is also identified when the child resisting contact with the alienated parent starts to enjoy parenting time and relinquishes the resistance they were displaying at the start of the visit (f & Bernet, 2020, p. 550).

Moderate Parental Alienation

According to Baker (2007), the moderate type of PAS is more fearsome, and the children are described as having "some parental programming against the targeted parent" and may struggle with visitation. A moderate level of PA is identified when the child exhibits strong resistance to the suggestion of contact with their alienated parent and is constantly oppositional toward the TP during parenting time visits. However, there are occasionally a few moments of encouraging connection between the child and the alienated parent (Lorandos & Bernet, 2020, p. 550). A further example of moderate PAS is characterised as the child being exposed to a considerable level of parental programming from the AP (Baker, 2007, p. 22). This programming creates a substantial internal battle for the child when visiting an alienated parent (Baker, 2007, p. 22). In these cases, the child may have a relationship with their TP that is reasonably strong, and eventually, they settle and adapt to the visit (Baker, 2007).

Severe Parental Alienation

In cases experiencing severe levels of SPA, children are adamant in their hatred of the alienated TP, often refusing visits with them and threatening to run away if a visit is proposed (Baker, 2007). Children experiencing severe levels of PA often have an unhealthy, enmeshed alliance with the AP, sharing paranoid fantasies about the TP to the point where the child's relationship with the TP is destroyed (Baker, 2007). Friends and family may also notice that the child and AP may have an unhealthy alliance (Baker, 2007). The definition of severe parental alienation (SPA), according to Lorandos et al. (2013), involves children who persistently and adamantly refuse all contact with the TP to the extent that they may even run away or hide to avoid spending time with them. Within the SPA context, visitation may be impossible due to the children being incredibly hostile to the point where the children may become physically violent toward the supposedly hated parent (Baker, 2007).

Other ways of acting out may be present, designed to cause formidable grief to the parent visited by the alienated child (Baker, 2007). These levels can manifest in behaviours such as running away and hiding to avoid seeing the alienated parent and remaining defiant and oppositional if they are made to spend parenting time with them (Baker, 2007). In addition, some severely alienated children exhibit behaviours such as persisting in not seeing the alienated parent and stating that they do not want to partake in a relationship with them (Lorandos & Bernet, 2020, p. 550). "In many cases, the children's hostility has reached paranoid levels, that is, delusions of persecution and fears that they will be murdered in situations where there is absolutely no evidence that such will be the case" (Gardner, 2008, p. 2).

Appendix Five

The Baker Strategy Questionnaire

Please complete and send it back with your numbers 0 to 4 at the end of each question.

Please rate each item on a 5-point Likert scale ranging from 0 (*never*) to 4 (*very often*).

One or both of my parents;

1. Made comments to me that fabricated or exaggerated the other parent's negative qualities while rarely saying anything positive about that parent; (Example, 2).
2. Limited or interfered with my contact with the other parent such that I spent less time with him/her than I was supposed to or could have;
3. Withheld or blocked phone messages, letters, cards, or gifts from the other parent meant for me;
4. Made it difficult for me and the other parent to reach and communicate with each other;
5. Indicated discomfort/displeasure when I spoke/asked about or had pictures of the other parent;

6. Became upset, cold, or detached when I showed affection for or spoke positively about the other parent;
7. Said and/or implied that the other parent did not really love me;
8. Created situations in which it was likely or expected that I choose him/her and reject the other parent;
9. Said things that indicated that the other parent was dangerous or unsafe;
10. Confided in me about "adult matters" that I probably should not have been told about (such as marital concerns or financial disputes), which led me to feel protective of him/her or angry at the other parent;
11. Created situations in which I felt obligated to show favouritism toward him/her and reject or rebuff/ignore the other parent;
12. Asked me to spy on or secretly obtain information from or about the other parent and report back to him/her;
13. Asked me to keep secrets from the other parent about things the other parent should have been informed about (e.g., upcoming plans, my whereabouts, etc.);
14. Referred to the other parent by his/her first name and appeared to want me to do the same;
15. Referred to his/her new spouse as Mom/Dad and appeared to want me to do the same;
16. Encouraged me to rely on his/her opinion and approval above all else;
17. Encouraged me to disregard/think less of the other parent's rules, values, and authority;

18. Made it hard for me or made me feel bad about spending time with the other parent's extended family;
19. Created situations in which it was likely that I would be angry with or hurt by the other parent.

Appendix Six

Semi-Structured Interview Schedule (Adult Survivors of SPA) Survey Questions

1. How many times have you accessed therapy for SPA from a mental health practitioner?
2. Was cost a contributing factor to your continuing/discontinuing therapy? If so, how and why?
3. Have you found a practitioner who understands SPA, and were they able to help you?
4. What types of therapy were tried or suggested by the practitioner to help you with your SPA symptoms?
5. Do you feel that this therapy/therapies helped you?
6. Can you describe how the therapy/therapies helped you as a client?
7. Can you describe why the therapy/therapies did not help you as a client?
8. How do you think your experience with therapy could have been improved?
9. Was the experience with the mental health practitioner positive or negative, or a combination?

10. Can you please elaborate on your experience with the practitioner?
11. Did the practitioner seem knowledgeable about SPA?
12. If they did seem knowledgeable about SPA, how did that feel for you?
13. How did that feel for you if they didn't seem knowledgeable about SPA?
14. What type of therapy/treatment do you think would be beneficial that you have not tried and why?
15. How would you describe yourself before accessing therapy/support?
16. How would you describe yourself after accessing therapy/support?
17. What other programs or ideas do you think could be developed to help other adult survivors of SPA?
18. What advice could you give to help more practitioners to understand the mind of an adult survivor of SPA?
19. Do you have anything that you would like to add regarding therapy for adult survivors of SPA?

Appendix Seven

Expression of Interest Flyer (Adult Survivors of SPA)

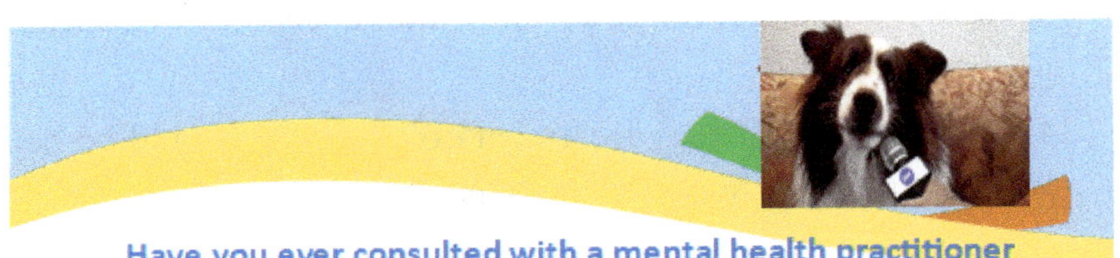

Have you ever consulted with a mental health practitioner about your parents high conflict divorce experienced as a child or adolescent?

Are you over 21 years of age?

If 'yes', then please read on...

If you identify as an adult child of high conflict divorce, otherwise known as severe parental alienation (SPA) and have spoken to a mental health practitioner about it, then we would like to hear from you.

We are interested in your experience of speaking with a mental health practitioner about the issue of SPA. If you would like to share this experience with us, research will be conducted as an informal interview, lasting approximately 60 to 90 minutes.

This is a great opportunity for you to contribute to furthering the education and practices of mental health practitioners, which may lead to an improvement in front line supports and services to other adult of SPA.

If you would like to participate in this study, or would like further information, then please contact the Student Researcher Alyse Price-Tobler on email alyse.price-tobler@research.usc.edu.au and leave a contact number (if in Australia) and a convenient time to be contacted.

Please note, Participation is subject to the number of expressions of interest, suitability and availability. This study is solely about your experience with mental health practitioners and not about your actual experience with severe parental alienation. Privacy and confidentiality is strictly adhered to in accordance with ethical guidelines. Thankyou.

Appendix Ten

Human Research Ethics Approval for Research Project

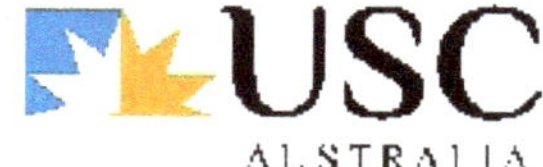

21 December 2021

A/Prof Andrew Crowden
Chair, Human Research Ethics Committee
Tel: +61 7 5430 2823
Email: humanethics@usc.edu.au

Dr Dyann Ross
Dr Peter Innes
Ms Alyse Price-Tobler
Dr Mandy Matthewson

Dear Investigators

Human research ethics approval for research project: Working with Adult Survivors of Severe Parental Alienation: Survivors and Mental Health Practitioners Perspective. A Qualitative Study (S211642)

This letter is to confirm that the USC Human Research Ethics Committee (HREC) has reviewed and granted ethics approval for this project subject to the standard conditions of approval listed below.

The period of ethics approval is from 21 December 2021 to 21 December 2024. The ethics approval number for the project is S211642. This number should be quoted on your Research Project Information Sheet and in any written communication with participants.

Ethics approval indicates that this project meets the requirements of the National Health and Medical Research Council's (NHMRC) *National Statement on Ethical Conduct in Human Research (2007)*. This does not negate the need for other approvals where relevant. It is the investigators' responsibility to ensure that all approvals relevant to this project are obtained.

If you have any queries or if you require further information, please contact us using the details above.

Yours sincerely

for
A/Prof Andrew Crowden
Chair, Human Research Ethics Committee

End of the thesis.

Abstract

In volume one, adult survivors provide insights into previously unexplored perspectives and experiences of complex intersecting traumas (CITs) associated with SPA. These include related parallel traumas such as child abduction, suicide, child filicide, and familicide, as well as family and domestic violence, psychological safety, prohibitive costs of therapy, identity issues, false allegations of child sexual abuse and domestic violence, persecutory delusions, abduction trauma, health literacy, and healing. Additionally, links between cancer and autoimmune disease, as well as a newly discovered 'specific phobia and anxiety variant', are addressed in this volume.

It is crucial to recognise that these courageous individuals are undertaking a journey to disrupt the intergenerational trauma patterns inherited from their ancestors. By engaging in this 'journey work,' they are actively transforming their lives to prevent future generations from enduring similar suffering. They stand as resilient warriors in the battle against child psychological and physical abuse.

www.ingramcontent.com/pod-product-compliance
Lightning Source LLC
Chambersburg PA
CBHW071324210326
41597CB00015B/1337

9781923087149